WENDY SAVAGE was born in South London in 1935. Educated at Croydon High School for Girls and Girton College, Cambridge, she started her clinical training at the London Hospital Medical College in East London in 1957. In 1962 she moved to Boston with her family where she worked as a research assistant at Boston City Hospital and gave birth to her third child. In 1964 her husband's job took the family to Nigeria where she learnt surgery and obstetrics and decided to specialise in obstetrics and gynaecology. Evacuated from Nigeria because of the outbreak of the Biafran war, Wendy Savage moved to Kenya where she worked as a Senior House Officer and then Registrar in Obstetrics and Gynaecology and then Surgery at Kenyatta National Hospital. On her return to England in 1969 she passed the examination for membership of the Royal College of Obstetricians and Gynaecologists (RCOG) and then left her job at the Royal Free Hospital to work in areas which she felt were neglected in orthodox training, such as family planning and venereal disease. At the same time she worked with the Pregnancy Advisory Service for a year as a counselling doctor and gynaecologist. In 1973 she left England for New Zealand with her four children where she worked for three years as a specialist in obstetrics, gynaecology, venereology and family planning, and gave evidence to the New Zealand Royal Commission on Contraception, Sterilisation and Abortion. In 1976 she returned to England to the London Hospital Medical College to work first as Lecturer and then, since August 1977, as Senior Lecturer and Honorary Consultant in Obstetrics and Gynaecology at the London Hospital. She was suspended from her clinical work there on 24 April 1985 until four and a half months after the public enquiry into her competence, held in February 1986, which exonerated her. On 24 July 1986 she was reinstated. She was elected a Fellow of the Royal College of Obstetricians and Gynaecologists in June 1985 and is the author of several medical publications, including three women's health books. Since 1978 she has been Press Officer for Doctors for a Woman's Choice on Abortion (DWCA). She lives in London with the youngest of her four children.

A
SAVAGE
ENQUIRY
Who Controls Childbirth?

· *Wendy Savage* ·

Published by VIRAGO PRESS Limited 1986
41 William IV Street, London WC2N 4DB

Copyright © Wendy Savage 1986

British Library Cataloguing in Publication Data

Savage, Wendy
  A Savage enquiry.
  1. Obstetrics
  I. Title
  618.2'092'4   RG524

ISBN 0-86068-859-3

Typeset by Rowland Phototypesetting Ltd,
Bury St Edmunds, Suffolk
Printed in Great Britain by Cox and Wyman Ltd,
Reading, Berkshire

· CONTENTS ·

To all those who have known doubt, perplexity and fear
as I have known them,
To all who have made mistakes as I have,
To all those whose humility increases with their knowledge
of this most fascinating subject,

THIS BOOK IS DEDICATED

Ian Donald wrote this dedication when he was Regius Professor of
Midwifery at the University of Glasgow for his book *Practical Obstetric
Problems* (Lloyd Luke 1955).
When I was working in Nigeria in 1964–7 his book was invaluable and I
was delighted and honoured when he gave me permission to use his
words for this book.
I think myself fortunate when I worked in Nairobi from 1967–9 to have
been trained by Glaswegians, as in general the Scottish contribution to
obstetrics has been notable, and in particular Ian Donald's immense
clinical knowledge has been complemented by his pioneering work with
ultrasound.

AND IN ADDITION

This book is dedicated to the women of the world who face the
uncertainty of childbirth with such optimism and courage.

· ACKNOWLEDGEMENTS ·

This book would not have been written without the assistance and friendship of Jane Leighton who, as a socialist and feminist, understood the medico-political issues so well; the support and enthusiasm of Debbie Owen, and the flexibility and encouragement of all the Virago staff. Brian Raymond has read numerous drafts rapidly and efficiently, and given me suggestions for more elegant phrases. Judi Dooling, Marianne Kilchenman and Barbara Smith have helped with some of the typing and Jane Hawksley redrafted chapter 2. I would like to thank them all for their help.

My thanks also to all those who have read parts of the manuscript and made suggestions comprehensively and fast despite their busy lives: Eva Alberman, Beverley Beech, Alex Campbell, Iain Chalmers, Peter Dunn, Myra Garrett, Sue Hadley, Marion Hall, Marky Hayton, John and Pauline Hendy, Edmund Hey, Peter Huntingford, Tony Jewell, James McGarry, John McGarry, Collette O'Neill, Heather Reid, David Ritchie, Christine Smith, Gordon Stirrat, Alec Turnbull, Sid Watkins, David Widgery. Some of their ideas and changes I have incorporated, but any inaccuracies are my responsibility and the sentiments are my own.

Brian Raymond encouraged me to start writing, and I would like to thank him and all those others who have made it possible to write this account of what was an important event in my life, but one which has far-reaching implications beyond myself.

I have had such strong and continuing support from too many people to name all of them individually, but I would like particularly to thank Luke Zander and Ron Taylor whose understanding of the principles of justice and own personal integrity have been an example to all doctors, and Sheila Hillier, Eva Alberman, Helen Bender, Alyson Hall, Irene Leigh, Colin Murray-Parkes, Frances Marks, Graeme Snodgrass, and Elizabeth Watson of the London Hospital and Medical College whose personal confidence in me has helped enormously. My thanks, too, to Mary Edmondson, Erica Jones, John Robson, Kambiz Boomla, Jane Taylor, Jo Shawcross, Liz Hodgetts, Alex Mills, Viv Taylor, Roseanna Pollen, Anna

Livingstone, Tom Kalloway, Bernard Taylor and Michael Liebson and all the other Tower Hamlets GPs who, with the midwives, in particular Jane Grant and Debbie Hughes, have worked so hard for my reinstatement and expressed their trust in me long before I was cleared.

Sheila Kitzinger and Iain Chalmers as well as providing moral support helped me with references, and the librarians at the Royal College of Obstetricians and Gynaecologists and all the library staff at the London Hospital Medical College have been efficient and sympathetic.

Phillipa Micklethwaite as President of the National Childbirth Trust, Beverley Beech of AIMS, Ruth Evans of the Maternity Alliance and Ron Brewer, Secretary of the Tower Hamlets CHC, have all been very helpful. The Support Group have worked immensely hard, and Sue Hadley, Heather Reid and Myra Garrett deserve special thanks. The Appeal Fund Committee did enormously well to raise over £60,000 for my legal costs and deal with the press whilst many of them were coping with young families as well as demanding jobs. I am sad that Sam Smith, who worked so hard, died a week after the enquiry finished and so missed the end of the story. My thanks to them all, and also the hundreds of people who have written to me, sent me cards and flowers and books, and the thousands who donated money and signed the petition presented to the DHSS.

Katy Simmons, Bob Moore, Joseph Winceslaus, Felicity Challoner, Alison Spankie, Melanie Davies, John MacVicar, Michael Moore and Mary McNabb were amongst those who gave affidavits for the High Court case and I am grateful to them for doing this at such short notice.

I would also like to thank the expert witnesses who appeared on my behalf at the enquiry, and gave hours of their precious time. They and my lawyers did this freely, and took on the task of defending me with no guarantee of payment, because of the principles involved.

I am grateful to the journalists in all the different types of media who have followed the case with interest and informed people about the issues; the MPs who have supported me in the House of Commons and outside; the many organisations who have publicised the struggle in their newsletters, and the unions and constituency Labour Parties, CHCs and women's groups who have spread the news and often sent contributions.

Lastly, I would like to thank my children for their support and understanding, in particular Wendy who kept my press-cuttings up to date, and Jay who bore the brunt of the phone calls and my preoccupation with the fight, and also the man who, like them, never doubted my competence – and whose advice and loving help (which included the meals I had not time to cook) kept me going during the lonely struggle before my suspension in April 1985.

Wendy Savage
Islington, 1 August 1986

· DRAMATIS PERSONAE ·

TOWER HAMLETS HEALTH AUTHORITY

Chairman	*Francis Cumberlege*
District Administrator till December 1985	*Sotiris Argyrou*
District Medical Officer	*Jean Richards**
District General Manager from 3.2.86	*John Alway*

PANEL OF ENQUIRY

Chairman	*Mr Christopher Beaumont*
Professor of Obstetrics and Gynaecology in Dundee	*Peter Howie*
Consultant Obstetrician and Gynaecologist, Rugby	*Leonard Harvey*

LAWYERS

Regional Legal Adviser till 30.6.86	*Terry Dibley*
Counsel for Tower Hamlets Health Authority	*Ian Kennedy QC*
	James Badenoch
Barrister instructed by the Medical Protections Society representing all the London Hospital doctors who gave evidence at the enquiry	*Mr Conlin*
Solicitors for Wendy Savage till 28.5.85	*James Watt* and *MAMS Leigh* of Hempsons
From June 1986 – present	*Brian Raymond* of Bindman and Partners
Counsel for Wendy Savage	*John Hendy*
Medico-legal expert retained by Hempsons	*Professor Geoffrey Chamberlain,* St Georges Hospital

LONDON HOSPITAL MEDICAL COLLEGE (LHMC)

Dean January 1983 to 30.9.86	*Mike Floyer*, Professor of Medicine*
Professor of Surgery to 30.9.85 and Dean July 1981 to December 1982	*David Ritchie*
Chairman of the Academic Division of Surgery	*John Blandy*, Professor of Urology*

Chairman of the Academic Board 1.10.85 to 30.9.86:	*Harry Allred,* Professor of Dentistry and Dean of Dental Studies. DHA member
Chairman of the Final Medical Committee and Medical Council	
February 1982 – January 1985	*Sid Watkins,* Professor of Neurosurgery
February 1985 – present	*Sam Cohen,* Professor of Psychiatry*

LONDON HOSPITAL

Department of Obstetrics and Gynaecology

Senior Consultant	*John Hartgill**
Chairman of the Division of Obstetrics and Gynaecology	*Trevor Beedham**
Consultant	*David Oram*
Senior Registrar	*Paul Armstrong*
Registrars	*Toby Fay, Hani Youssef, Gillian Robinson*

Department of Paediatrics

| Senior Lecturer in Paediatrics | *Roger Harris* |

JOINT APPOINTMENTS LHMC AND ST BARTHOLOMEW'S MEDICAL COLLEGE

Professor of Obstetrics and Gynaecology	*Jurgis Gediminis Grudzinskas (Gedis)* Based at LHMC and London Hospital
Professor of Reproductive Physiology	*Tim Chard.* Based at Bart's
Senior Lecturer in Obstetrics and Gynaecology	*Wendy Savage.* Based at LHMC and London Hospital (Mile End)*
Lecturer in Obstetrics and Gynaecology	*Tony Nysenbaum*
Professor of Clinical Epidemiology	*Eva Alberman.* Based at LHMC*

ST BARTHOLOMEW'S HOSPITAL

| Senior Consultant in Obstetrics and Gynaecology until December 1985 | *Gordon Bourne,* Regional Assessor in Obstetrics for North East Thames Region. Expert witness at the enquiry in February 1986 |

GENERAL PRACTITIONERS IN TOWER HAMLETS

Dr Sam Smith, retired. Founder of St Stephens Road practice. Treasurer of Appeal Fund*

Mary Edmondson, General Practitioner Obstetrician (GPO), Steele's Lane Health Centre. Secretary of Appeal Fund

Tony Jewell, GPO, South Poplar practice. TUC nominee on the DHA. Chair of Appeal Fund*

WENDY SAVAGE SUPPORT CAMPAIGN

| Chair | *Beverley Beech* of Association for Improvements in the Maternity Services (AIMS) and Health Rights |
| Vice-Chair | *Ron Brewer,* Secretary of the Community Health Council (CHC) |

· Dramatis Personae ·

| Members of Executive Committee | *Sue Hadley* and *Heather Reid* of National Childbirth Trust (NCT), *Myra Garrett* of Tower Hamlets Health Campaign (THHC), *Kate Parkin*, *Lucy Micklethwaite* |
| Other Supporters | *Luke Zander*, Senior Lecturer in General Practice, St Thomas's, *Sheila Kitzinger*, anthropologist, author and natural childbirth teacher |

EXPERT WITNESSES CALLED BY THE HEALTH AUTHORITY: 'THE PROSECUTION'

John Dennis: Professor of Obstetrics and Gynaecology, Southampton, Regional Assessor in Obstetrics for Wessex

Gordon Bourne: see above

EXPERT WITNESSES CALLED BY WENDY SAVAGE: 'THE DEFENCE'

Peter Dunn: Reader in Child Health, University of Bristol

Alexander Campbell: Professor of Paediatrics, University of Aberdeen

Iain Chalmers: Director of the National Perinatal Epidemiology Unit

Marion Hall: Consultant Obstetrician and Gynaecologist and Honorary Senior Lecturer, University of Aberdeen

Edmund Hey: Consultant Paediatrician, Newcastle

James McGarry: Consultant Obstetrician and Gynaecologist and Honorary Clinical Lecturer, University of Glasgow

John McGarry: Consultant Obstetrician and Gynaecologist, North Devon District Hospital, Barnstaple

Gordon Stirrat: Professor of Obstetrics and Gynaecology, University of Bristol

Ron Taylor: Professor of Obstetrics and Gynaecology, United Medical School of St Thomas's and Guys', London

* denotes a graduate of the London Hospital Medical College

1984–1985

Connections between Tower Hamlets Health Authority & London Hospital Medical College

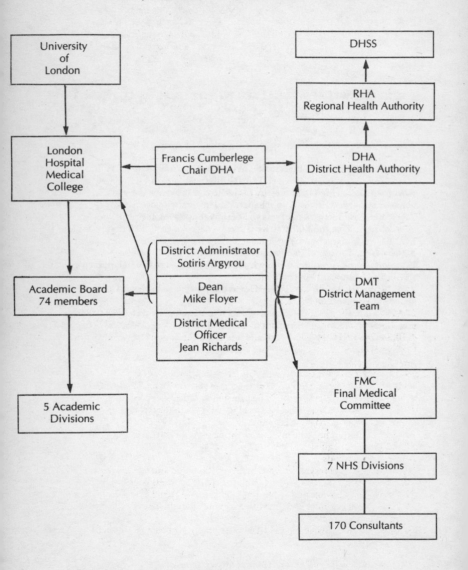

· CHRONOLOGY ·

August 1977 Wendy Savage appointed Senior Lecturer in Peter Huntingford's department
July 1981 Peter Huntingford leaves. Trevor Beedham appointed
Jan 1983 Gedis Grudzinskas and David Oram appointed
Jan 1984 District Health Authority decide to centralise obstetric and gynaecological services at Whitechapel
20.2.84 and **19.3.84** Grudzinskas writes to Wendy Savage re employment
26.4.84 Baby U born. **3.5.84** Baby U dies
21.5.84 Trevor Beedham's letter to Gedis Grudzinskas which served as a formal request to the District Administrator for an enquiry into the U case.
21.8.84 Wendy Savage notified by District Administrator of Us' formal complaint through Community Health Council
24.9.84 Wendy Savage and Roger Harris see Us with secretary of Community Health Council
27.9.84 Jean Richards, District Medical Officer, mentions HM (61)112 and possibility of sending U case notes to Gordon Bourne
4.10.84 and **12.10.84** Wendy Savage sees Dean of London Hospital Medical College, who tells her: 'One case not enough for a 112'
24.4.85 Suspended
13.6.85 March on District Health Authority in protest
28.6.85 Wendy Savage replies to criticisms of cases to Chairman of DHA
5.8.85 High Court application to be heard in vacation accepted
15.8.85 Decision taken to proceed to HM (61)112 enquiry, communicated to Wendy Savage's lawyers, Bindmans
2.9.85 High Court judge turns down hearing for a breach of contract
3.2.86 Enquiry begins
8.3.86 Enquiry ends
9.7.86 First part of report received by Brian Raymond and Wendy Savage
10.7.86 Second March organised by Support Group, press conference
21.7.86 Wendy Savage and Brian Raymond receive Part 2 of report
24.7.86 Towers Hamlet Health Authority vote unanimously to reinstate Wendy Savage, Cumberlege holds press conference
10.10.86 Wendy Savage returns to work as practising obstetrician and gynaecologist

· Introduction ·

She should have been a good and agreeable girl and made sure
she got on with her colleagues. If she had played her cards right
she would have found being a woman was to her advantage and
her male colleagues might have been prepared to do her
more favours.

Senior obstetrician quoted in *Sunday Times*, 9 March 1986

I was suspended from my post as Honorary Consultant in Obstetrics and Gynaecology to the Tower Hamlets Health Authority on 24 April 1985, on the grounds of alleged incompetence, after twenty-five years in medical practice. I realised then what millions of other people in this country already know – that the loss of your job is a shattering experience. I was lucky not to have to share their financial anxieties, as I was suspended on full pay as Senior Lecturer in Obstetrics and Gynaecology at the London Hospital Medical College; but the allegation of professional incompetence, and the abrupt ending of my active role of looking after patients and teaching students, was devastating.

The loss of my job was like a bereavement. Powerful, confusing and shifting emotions swept over me – disbelief (can this really be happening?), sadness, guilt, self-doubt, anger.

Attempting to deal with these emotions in a totally unfamiliar situation – as a client of lawyers, a person responding to events over which she has no control – was a sharp contrast to my usual role of the autonomous doctor, making daily decisions close to life and death; an independent woman in command of her own world. The added and unsought responsibility of responding to media attention and finding that I had become a public figure, a spokesperson for the pregnant woman, has not been easy. It has only been possible because of the immense support I have had. That support has helped me to sustain my inner conviction that I must fight back and win this battle, not only for myself but for all women.

Over the years I have been practising, I have learnt that women need to be able to talk as equals with doctors, to be informed of the choices available to them and encouraged to make up their own minds about becoming pregnant, or continuing with a pregnancy. I have realised how important it is for a woman to feel in control of the birth process if she is going to emerge as a confident parent. I have become increasingly aware of the deficiencies in the care that we, as obstetricians, provide for pregnant women.

Pregnancy is not an illness. I belong to the school of thought which believes that every pregnancy is normal unless there are indications that something is wrong. Those at the opposite end of the obstetric spectrum believe that no pregnancy is normal, except in retrospect. This attitude, together with the labelling of women as high risk on the basis of statistical, rather than individual information, leads to a situation where too many women are forced to attend hospital clinics, rather than having the more personal care of the midwife or a general practitioner closer to home. I feel that as the risks in childbirth become smaller, statistical methods of predicting (on the basis of her age, number of children or income) which woman will lose her baby have limited use. In my view, if you look at each woman as an individual, and plan her care with her, you will get the best result.

I and many of my supporters saw my suspension as part of the continuing struggle about who controls childbirth, and it was on this ground that we chose to fight. It was only about the issues of choices in childbirth that I was prepared to speak publicly, but at a deeper level, I knew that this battle was about the way doctors relate to and work with each other, and about the fact that I am not a member of the 'establishment' and saw no reason to conform to the medical profession's unwritten, but well understood 'party line', especially if I thought this was not in the interests of patients.

These issues do not lend themselves to the shorthand, confrontational approach of the media, and at first I felt they were best resolved privately. Up to the time that the enquiry started in February 1986 I hoped, somewhat idealistically, that it would be possible to accomplish this. But the aggressive way that the Health Authority case was conducted, the initial response of my accusers in the face of the expert opinions of obstetricians and paediatricians who supported my disputed management, and the report of the panel which exonerated me, have convinced me that the medical politics which underlie my suspension need to be revealed.

This book has been written for a number of reasons. First, so that my supporters can fill in the gaps in the story which they followed in the newspapers, and to express my gratitude for their trust in me and what I was fighting for.

Second, although I know it will upset many members of the medical profession, who feel we should not wash our dirty linen in public, I hope that doctors who read this will understand that the actions of my colleagues at the London Hospital were not significantly different from those taking place every week in other hospitals and medical academic units in this country. I believe such behaviour arises from the way we, as a profession, have organised ourselves. We also need to look closely at what it is in the training of doctors and the institutions we have set up – the British Medical Association, the Royal Colleges, the General Medical Council – which made it so difficult for the leaders of our profession to act effectively against the injustice of my suspension, despite the immediate, strongly expressed support from local patients and GPs. We need to make positive changes in the regulations for disciplining doctors which will prevent a repetition of the damaging, prolonged, bitter and expensive battle which has taken place over the last fifteen months. I hope that my colleagues at the London Hospital will accept this as a constructive attempt to understand the issues and actions which lay behind my suspension.

Third, for myself, there is a need to work through, and make sense of, this extraordinary experience. Right at the start I made the decision that I was not going to conduct myself as a 'guilty' person because I knew that the charge was false. I was going to carry on going into work, doing teaching and research as far as possible and accept invitations to talk about obstetrics and gynaecology as if there was no threat to my professional livelihood or slur on my reputation hanging over me. I hope, by sharing this ordeal with others, that I will be able to put the horrific part of these fifteen months behind me, and take forward the good things: the trust, friendship and generosity of those who have supported me.

25 July 1986

· CHAPTER 1 ·

Suspension

'Now for the evidence,' said the King, 'and then the sentence.'
'No!' said the Queen, 'first the sentence, and then the evidence!'
'Nonsense!' cried Alice, so loudly that everybody jumped, 'the
idea of having the sentence first!'

Lewis Carroll, *Alice's Adventures under Ground*

Tuesday, 23 April 1985
A telephone call interrupts my gynaecology clinic at Mile End
Hospital. I am seeing the ninth of the fifteen women booked for this
morning. She is about my age – fifty – with a common problem for
women approaching the menopause. She thought her periods had
stopped and then, a year later, she had some bleeding. Women
know that this may be a sign of cancer and it is always difficult for
the doctor both to allay their fears and yet do the necessary D and
C (dilation and curettage – scraping of the inside of the womb to
make sure there is no abnormal growth there). I am listening to the
woman and am irritated to be interrupted at a delicate stage of the
consultation by a nurse saying that Dr Richards is on the telephone
and wants to make an appointment to see me. I ask her to tell Dr
Richards the times when I will be available and resume the
conversation.

We try to create as much privacy as possible at the Mile End
clinic. If the woman agrees to a medical student being present at
her consultation, we allow a single student to attend. If she does
not want a medical student present we respect her wishes. This
woman has agreed, and I am trying to show the medical student
how to pass a speculum, an instrument which is inserted into the
vagina to look at the neck of the womb; this is a task which requires
some skill and about which the woman often feels quite embarrassed. The nurse returns and tells me that Dr Richards insists on
speaking to me herself. I apologise to the woman lying on the
consulting room couch, walk into the reception area, pick up the
telephone and suggest Thursday. Jean replies: 'That's no good,
because I am going to suspend your clinical contract tomorrow.'

1

I hear myself arranging to meet her at 6.30 p.m. the next day, walk past the clerks and the crowded waiting room, back to the consulting room and book an operation date for the patient. After she has dressed I explain, as if in a dream, what the operation involves. As she leaves, the registrar comes in for the operating diary. He takes one look at my face and asks me what is wrong. I do not tell him I am to be suspended. I've never heard of a doctor being suspended before, except for madness. On the verge of tears, I tell him only that I have heard from Jean Richards, the District Medical Officer, that my Professor of Obstetrics, Gedis Grudzins-kas, has taken the case notes of some of my patients without my knowledge and these have been sent, with critical comments, to Gordon Bourne, the Regional Assessor for Maternal Mortality. His reply shocks me: 'I knew that Trevor Beedham [a fellow obstetrician] was gunning for you, but I didn't know about the professor.'

Elizabeth, the nurse, brings me coffee and I pull myself together and see the rest of the women booked for the clinic. There are moments when a woman's problems make me forget my own, but later I cannot recall who I have seen. For once, I finish the clinic on time.

As it happens, I already have an appointment with Mike Floyer, the Dean of the London Hospital Medical College, at one o'clock. I have asked to see him because last Friday I heard Jean Richards upsetting my secretary by demanding case notes of patients in my care. 'To send to Gordon Bourne,' she said, when I questioned her. I replied, 'Christ, Jean, if the professor thinks he's going to get rid of me I'll fight him every inch of the way.'

Driving through the back streets of London's East End to see the dean at the main hospital, I recall that Jean had mentioned Gordon Bourne's name a few months earlier, in September 1984, when an investigation was being considered into a case where I had allowed a woman whose baby was in the breech position to try a natural labour. But although I have seen Jean about every six weeks or so since then, she has never mentioned the matter again.

As I walk from the consultants' car park, past Queen Alexandra's statue in the garden of the hospital, I wonder what has been happening behind the scenes between September and April.

Along the corridor to the dean's office I notice, as I always notice, the rows of photographs of men who have taught medicine

2

there. I remember the impact this phalanx of serious middle-aged faces had on me when I first came here twenty-eight years ago to be interviewed for entry to medical school. I sit, as I did then, on the hard leatherette sofa, and tell myself that I must keep calm; and above all I must not cry.

Mike is his usual friendly self. His gangling, rather vague appearance fits his reputation for 'patent honesty'. I find myself starting to speak before he offers me one of the low armchairs. 'I made this appointment because it's becoming impossible to work with the professor. But Jean Richards has just told me that she is going to suspend my Honorary Consultant contract tomorrow.' Mike, whom I had always trusted, shows no shock, surprise or sympathy. Calmly, he tells me that he was present at the meeting, five days ago, when the Chairman of Tower Hamlets Health Authority, its legal adviser, the District Medical Officer and the District Administrator decided to suspend me.

How can such a decision be taken without my knowledge? Mike replies, 'The professor should have told you. I rather thought he had . . . the college will go on paying you, but whether you carry on with your student teaching will depend on the professor. I don't know enough about obstetrics to argue about the decision.' I ask him what will happen to my patients while I am suspended. Mike says he supposes that the professor will look after them.

I drive to the GPs' surgery in St Stephen's Road for my antenatal clinic. It is a busy clinic. Between seeing the women I telephone lawyers and an administrator friend. During the clinic, Tony Jewell, a GP who is the TUC nominee on the District Health Authority, rings me. His wife is due to have her second baby under my care in three weeks' time. I tell him the news, swear him to silence and say that I hope I can get something done to stop this before tomorrow afternoon. After the clinic I return to Mile End to dictate the letters from the gynae clinic that morning. Usually I have all the details of the women in my mind and I merely have to glance at the folder in order to dictate the letter. But tonight I have to read through all the notes before recalling each patient. I leave about half-past eight and eat with a friend. I feel dazed and am unable to taste the food.

Wednesday, 24 April 1985
At 4 a.m. I awake suddenly and completely. This is so unjust, so

outrageous, there must be some way it can be stopped. I write a letter to the Medical Defence Union which, with the Medical Protection Society, is an organisation to which doctors must subscribe for the protection of their legal interests. Can we take out an injunction? In the early morning light I drive along the empty London streets to Harley Street and push the letter, marked URGENT, through the elegant door of the MDU in Devonshire Place.

After the morning antenatal clinic comes the ward and necessary excuses to the women in my care. One has been admitted several times with pelvic infection and is due to have a laparoscopy to see whether her tubes are damaged. I have to tell her that my registrar will do the operation. She looks disappointed and is surprised by my change of plan. It is not that the operation is hard to do, but I know her and she has trusted me through several difficult years, and I had promised to do the operation myself. We always organise our lists so that the doctor who sees the woman in outpatients does the operation. It makes so much difference to women when they already know the doctor who is to do the operation – it also makes mistakes less likely to occur. I almost break down as I sit on the bed to tell another woman who has lost two babies that I can no longer care for her.

I meet five of the junior staff in my office. In confidence I tell them about my suspension, now only minutes away; I ask them to look after the patients and we talk over the outstanding problems.

I drive numbly to the administrative headquarters in the main hospital at Whitechapel to keep the appointment with Jean Richards. The Medical Defence Union have arranged for a solicitor to meet me at the front door. He looks awfully young.

I tell the solicitor what has happened as we walk up the narrow stairs to the top floor where Jean has her office. Jean, a few years older than me, also trained at the London Hospital. Business-like, she hands me the papers relating to my suspension, explaining to the solicitor that I am being charged with professional incompetence. As I check the documents, we discuss things calmly, even amicably. I am more concerned with arrangements for the care of my patients. The solicitor says: 'You seem like old friends.' Jean replies, 'We are, we've known each other for twenty-five years.'

Thursday, 25 April 1985

Again, I wake at 4 a.m. Rereading the suspension documents, which cite five cases in which my management of labour is said to give rise to serious concern about the safety of patients in my care, I think: this isn't about competence, it's about attitudes, about a different approach to maternity care.

The strange thought that I am not to be allowed into theatre preoccupies me during the three mile drive from home to Mile End Hospital. Jean telephones me, reminding me that I must leave my office and offers transport to move my belongings. I begin to pack up my papers, make telephone calls, dictate letters. Just before two o'clock, the professor comes to see me. Jurgis (also known as Gedis) Grudzinskas is forty years old, with striking blue eyes. His fair hair is beginning to recede a little. Although Australian by upbringing, his accent is mid-Atlantic. His usual friendly manner is replaced by a hurried formality. In four minutes precisely, he tells me that he learned about my suspension that morning, is cancelling my lecture scheduled for the afternoon, that I must leave my academic office in his department too, and am to be withdrawn from teaching. He hands me a letter of confirmation. His action provokes a strange response in me. A cold rage prevents me from speaking. And, inexplicably, my anger is mixed with pity for him.

I spend the rest of the day making arrangements for other people to deal with outstanding clinical problems. I am surprised to find that someone has already told my junior staff that five cases are involved. I reassure them that those who have been involved in the care of the five women should not be damaged by battles between consultants.

Friday, 26 April 1985

It feels unreal to be barred from working and cut off from my professional life. The loss, the sense of powerlessness increases when, simultaneously, I find myself delivered into the hands of another set of professionals, with a completely different language and way of working – the lawyers.

The solicitors instructed on my behalf by the MDU, Hempsons, have their offices in Henrietta Street in Covent Garden. The heavy wooden door with its brass plate leads to a worn, wooden staircase. The small waiting room has Regency chairs, *The Times* and vases of flowers. I sit there with some impatience and trepidation. After ten minutes I am taken across the street to the third floor of a newly decorated cream and brown Gothic building which reminds me of an Oxbridge college.

I am expecting to see Mr Watt, with whom I have had dealings before, and am surprised to be greeted by another solicitor, who introduces himself as Mr Leigh. He is about thirty-five, good-looking, with a self-confident manner. As we size each other up I think: intelligent, quick to grasp the facts; but will he understand that I am not incompetent? This is a battle about the care of women, usually provided by men – and the law is dominated by men, too. I try to convince him that the situation will actually 'right itself' once the truth is known.

The press have already telephoned. I accept his advice not to make a public statement.

It is ten minutes past seven when I leave, grateful for having had the opportunity to talk. The usual office bustle has ceased and I walk rapidly to my car. As usual, I am a little behind schedule. I have to be at the medical students' dinner within an hour and must go home first. Threading my way through the tourists, I wryly think that I might manage to get to things on time in the next few months: I will no longer have to answer a telephone call as I leave the office for a meeting, or see the patients whose problems spill over from the morning to the afternoon clinic. As I unlock my front door, uncharacteristically thinking about what to wear that evening, it hits me. I don't have a working day any more. There will be no more calls in the middle of the night, no more driving through dark streets to see a labouring woman. I feel useless. All I can see is emptiness. Fortunately my sixteen-year-old son hears the key turning the lock. 'What's for supper? Are you being paid? So what's the problem?' I laugh and dash upstairs to change, wondering how I'm going to cope, facing all the people who know I am suspended, but won't know why.

· CHAPTER 2 ·

The Making of an Obstetrician

Women constitute half of the world's population, perform nearly two-thirds of its work hours, receive one-tenth of the world's income and own less than one hundredth of the world's property.

United Nations report, 1980

I did not start my medical career as a 'radical in the labour ward'. But my career as a doctor, like that of many women, has not followed an orthodox pattern. What I have learnt from being a doctor and a working mother in four continents, and what I have learnt from patients, is that women are individuals, and they should have control over their own fertility. Informed choice is a prerequisite for that control, and professional advisers who are prepared to share information and decision-making with the woman are essential.

I was born in 1935 and spent the first five years of my life in Norbury, a green and undistinguished suburb of South London. At the outbreak of the Second World War my father, who was working as a chartered surveyor, was called up and sent to Scotland. My mother and we children – I had a brother and sister by now – were evacuated to Horsham in Sussex.

When I was eight years old, my life changed completely. My mother died and we were sent to boarding school in Devon. After the war my father remarried. He bought a large Victorian house in Surrey cheaply, as the garden was pitted with bomb craters, and proceeded to rebuild the house and transform seven acres of a hawthorn and bramble wilderness into a beautiful garden. The idea that it was possible to change things physically and in an unorthodox way was firmly implanted in my mind as I sat on ladders to steady them while my father knocked down chimneys and walls, and dug out tons of chalk to create his garden.

I went to Croydon High School for Girls: a direct grant school, proud of its academic reputation, but also concerned to produce young women who were not just bluestockings but cared about people as well.

No one in my family had been to university. My father had left school at sixteen and educated himself at evening classes; so had his three sisters whose formal education finished even earlier, at thirteen or fourteen. He and one of my aunts had started their own businesses and all my aunts worked, two choosing not to have children.

I was not part of a class which accepted status and success as their due: my family was self-directing, hard-working and earned respect because of the quality of their work. I remember the feeling of independence when I got an exhibition to pay my fees in the sixth form and how privileged I felt to have the chance of a good education and, later, a profession. The example of my family's disciplined approach to work has remained a powerful influence in my own working life.

I went to Cambridge in 1953. There, for the first time in my life, I was discriminated against because of my sex. From the age of fourteen I had wanted to be a research chemist, but after a year of physics, chemistry, mineralogy and mathematics – and seeing how research chemists actually work – I decided I wanted more contact with people. One morning in the summer vacation I woke up knowing that I wanted to be a doctor.

Two men who had changed to medicine from classics and modern languages were allowed to learn three science subjects from scratch and complete their second MB, the initial stage of their medical degree, in three years. I had only to learn one new subject; but I had to wait a year for admission to the medical course because there was a quota for women students; my participation would have increased the number of women medical students by half a percent, to 10.5 per cent. So I had to spend a fourth year at Cambridge which I accepted philosophically; academically it was a fairly relaxed year. I took the opportunity to attend psychology and history of art lectures and hardly spoke to medical students because I was 'out of phase'. My father had not been pleased with my decision to do medicine and thought that three years of higher education was enough, so after I obtained my degree, my tutor found a grant for my fees.

I started clinical training at the London Hospital Medical College in the East End of London in October 1957, along with

three other women and about fifty men. Not as upper class as St
Thomas's, as intellectual as University College or quite so rugby-
oriented as St Mary's, the London Hospital Medical College
(founded in 1785, the first medical school in England) has always
had a tradition of service to the local community. An unusually
high number of graduates for a London college – about half – went
into General Practice, and it was comparatively progressive in its
attitude to women. In the fifties, other hospitals rarely appointed
women even to the most junior posts, but at the London women
had been known to become registrars! One of the three clinical
professors was a woman, Dorothy Russell, a distinguished neuropathologist.

As students, we were divided into groups of between six and
eight, and as we moved through the specialties in our second and
third years, we were attached to the teams of doctors which made
up a 'firm', and got to know each other well. I found the clinical
work with patients absorbing and enjoyable, although in some
specialties death was frighteningly close and the suffering of people
hard to bear.

In those days, before the 'rationalisation' of the health service,
the London Hospital was supported by a network of smaller
hospitals in the area now known as the London Borough of Tower
Hamlets. Most of our patients lived in Stepney, Bethnal Green,
Bow, Poplar, Wapping, Spitalfields and the Isle of Dogs, although
for the special departments they came from all over the East End of
London and Essex.

As a port area, East London has been the traditional entry point
of refugees, starting with the Huguenots who came to Spitalfields
to escape religious persecution after the Revocation of the Edict of
Nantes in 1685. Since the Huguenots, successive waves of immig-
rants have come to the East End, migrating out as they became
more prosperous. When I was a student, many of those living in the
vicinity of the London Hospital had come from Russia and Poland
at the turn of the century and still spoke only Yiddish. The shops in
Brick Lane, now filled with Halal meat, exotic vegetables and
spices, were then Kosher butchers, grocery stores with pickled
herrings and lox, and, a rarity outside the Whitechapel area in
those days, bakers selling bagels and good rye bread.

I lived, for the final year of my training, in a hospital house just
behind the outpatients. I could get out of bed at five to nine, dash

downstairs and be sitting in outpatients for nine o'clock. Two of my teachers, Dr Archie Clark-Kennedy and Dr Donald Hunter, made a deep impression on me. Dr Clark-Kennedy emphasised that one must see the person as a whole and understand their place in the world, as part of a family and a community, not just a 'patient' in a hospital bed. And I can still remember the passion with which Donald Hunter, who founded the specialty of industrial medicine, spoke on our ward rounds about the exploitation of workers, and the callous disregard of employers for safety regulations. I remember, too, his distaste for the way that some doctors in private practice behaved towards patients. He often quoted the great Canadian physician, Osler: 'Listen to the patient; he is telling you the diagnosis.'

When I did my obstetric training in 1958, we still had quite a large number of home deliveries. The district midwives had a house behind the Medical College on Turner Street from which they would issue forth on their bicycles with their black 'midder' bags strapped on the backs. They and the students were ruled firmly by Sister Gladys, who never seemed to have any time off. During our first month of midwifery we were not supposed to leave the premises either and were called in turn to look after women in labour, with whom we sat until they were delivered either in hospital or at home.

My first delivery was in the district. I had never even seen a film of a baby being born. An Irish woman was having her fourth baby in a flat in Blackwall Buildings. The midwife helped me through the delivery. 'Now,' she said, pretending she was speaking to the patient, 'Doctor is going to put on her gloves. Now, Doctor is going to do a vaginal examination, and she will be feeling where the head is, and whether the neck of the womb is still there.' (I had never felt either a baby's head or the neck of a womb before.) The woman wanted to push, and I could see some dark hair as the baby's head became visible. Another push; and suddenly there was this baby crying on the bed. I was astounded. It seemed so easy. I'd been brought up on *Gone with the Wind* and had expected agony and writhing and sweating as the woman pulled on knotted sheets. I often wonder whether the fact that my first experience of birth was so natural and relaxed has influenced my approach to obstetrics. Perhaps a doctor whose first experience is of seeing a Caesarean section has his or her view of the process of childbirth set by that experience, so that surgical rather than natural delivery seems the normal way to have a baby.

One experience which I will never forget was attending a fifteen-year-old girl at East Mount Street. She had concealed the pregnancy and had delivered a stillborn baby lying on an iron bedstead among dirty sheets in a bleak, carpetless room. I felt a numbed horror. It made me incapable of speech or any kind of helpful gesture towards the pale, thin girl with her dead baby lying silent between her legs. I will never forget the feeling of emptiness, which was mirrored by the cold house, her unfriendly and uncommunicative mother and the bare room with the iron bed.

The same feeling of emptiness struck me again later that month at another stillbirth. The woman had a malignant melanoma (a cancer of the skin) and they ruptured her membranes (broke her waters) to speed up the birth. It was obvious that something was wrong when the liquor (the fluid round the baby) shot right across the room, hitting the registrar. The midwife leant down to listen for the baby's heart beat, and I could tell from her face that it wasn't there. The liquor had come out too rapidly and the pressure changes had caused the placenta to separate from the uterine wall, cutting off the baby's oxygen supply. Suddenly, again, there was this awful feeling of emptiness in the room. Nobody said anything. But I knew, strongly and instinctively, that it was wrong not to tell the woman.

Obstetrics and Emotion

Those two stillbirths made a deep impression on me and have influenced my thinking on the way that doctors' own feelings, if unacknowledged, can block their ability to be of help to the patient.

Even today, despite a reduction in the perinatal mortality rate – death of babies between the seventh month of pregnancy and the first week of life – one woman in a hundred leaves hospital without a live baby, and in a unit delivering 3000 women a year, a perinatal death will occur every fortnight. But doctors still have difficulty in dealing with their own feelings about stillbirth. In 1970, an obstetrician named Pat Giles, a professor in Perth, Australia, studied forty women who had lost babies in the first week of life or as stillbirths, and said, 'Although doctors treated the women's physical symptoms and prescribed sedatives liberally, in about half the cases they avoided discussing the death of the baby.'

Later in my career, I began to note how women who had not delivered a live baby, or whose babies had died, were given a separate room, to spare their feelings, but often these rooms were missed out of the ward round. Students were not allocated to these women. They were discharged home as soon as medically possible, and if they failed to keep their postnatal appointment, there was a tendency to leave it at that. I had no idea what happened to the babies and apart from signing the stillbirth certificate and requesting a post-mortem, the doctor was not involved in thinking about the disposal of the body.

I remember vividly the first time (after nine years of obstetrics and over 100 perinatal deaths) that I asked a woman if she wanted to see her dead baby. The baby's skin was just beginning to peel and he had a forceps mark on one cheek. But I wrapped him up and carried him to his mother. 'Oh,' she said, 'isn't he beautiful.' The midwives had wanted to stop me, but they too realised, when they saw how naturally the woman held him, that what they had been taught needed to be changed.

Doctors have very little training, either formal or informal, in dealing with their own feelings of pain and sadness. Those who choose obstetrics enjoy their work because of the rewards of delivering women of healthy babies, and often feel a sense of failure when they cannot achieve this. In most British hospitals there is no support group for the house staff where they can discuss and explore their feelings. This will depend on the relationships between individual doctors and consultants which is hampered, often, by the hierarchical nature of the profession and the need for references within the career structure, so that it can be very difficult for a young doctor to openly admit what he or she is going through.

Doctors experience all the classic symptoms of grief – shock, denial, guilt and anger, but these are often only expressed in ways which make the death harder for the baby's mother to bear. Shocked, the doctor may appear callous as he blocks off his feelings in order to control the situation. Denial may be expressed by his or her inability to say plainly that the baby is dead, and by the use of artificial aids which hopelessly extend the 'life' of the baby in the intensive care unit. The pain and sadness is banished by discharging the woman early, and even by arranging for the postnatal examination to be done by her general practitioner. Anger and hostility may even extend to the woman herself, whose lack of antenatal attendance and failure to submit herself to tests may be censured.

If a doctor has made a mistake, his or her feeling of guilt may be overwhelming, and shame makes it difficult to admit errors. The lack of a suitable framework in most hospitals for doctors to admit these feelings and understand what is happening to themselves is, I think, responsible for the seemingly uncaring attitudes which some doctors develop.

The Birth of My Own Children

Most obstetricians see more abnormal deliveries than normal deliveries because normal deliveries will be dealt with almost entirely by the midwives. During the two months of my student obstetric training I did eighty-seven deliveries altogether, the largest cluster of normal deliveries with which I have been involved. It is still true today that the only time a doctor will see and spend time with straightforward deliveries is when he or she is a student.

Just after my finals I married and I had Yewande, my first baby, in the middle of my pre-registration year. I knew my husband Mike wanted to take a job abroad and that if I wanted to get registered before we left I had to get the time in, so after medical posts in Christchurch and Exeter, I offered my services to the London Hospital without pay. They made me stop work when I was thirty-six weeks pregnant, four weeks before the baby was due; then, of course, I was two weeks overdue! I was full of energy, and used the time to decorate the house. When my baby was five weeks old I got a paid job in the Receiving Room (Casualty), which was really the only possible post at the London for a woman with a baby in those days, when everyone worked through the weekends and every night and lived a (fairly) monastic life in the doctors' mess. In the RR we worked a shift system. We had one day a week off and worked nights, 11 p.m. to 9 a.m., for seven days every six weeks or so. I used to go home and breastfeed Yandy at lunchtime and she slept behind the RR in the doctors' room when I was on nights. The next year, pregnant again, I did a locum in general practice and worked until my estimated date of delivery, but again I was overdue and was induced at forty-two weeks by John Hartgill, then the middle registrar at the London Hospital and now the senior consultant there.

When my second daughter, Wendy, was three weeks old, we went to the United States. Mike had got a job in educational research in Boston, working out ways of teaching science to primary school children. There I got a job as a research assistant with Professor Ed Kass at Boston City Hospital, situated in one of the poorest parts of the city. It was an intellectually stimulating and happy department and I enjoyed learning about epidemiology and infectious disease.

Pregnant for the third time, I didn't fancy the epidural and forceps package then fashionable in the States and found an obstetrician who believed in normal delivery. Nicholas took five hours to be born, and I was sitting up and drinking coffee ten minutes later. The obstetrician turned to the nurses who had never seen a woman give birth without forceps before. 'That's natural childbirth,' he said.

Mike's job then took us to Nigeria, to Awo-omamma, a village in the east, where, in a small local hospital, I learnt surgery and obstetrics from an excellent Italian surgeon, Dr Angelo Caroli. When he went on a much needed holiday I found myself in charge, single-handed, of the small independent hospital. I quickly learned about management and finance, as well as how to face up to frightening uncertainty about the vast range of clinical conditions provided by the seventy-five patients

We next moved to Enugu, the capital of the eastern region of Nigeria, where I learned that women will risk death to rid themselves of an unwanted pregnancy. I was forcibly hit by the injustice of a health system where money is the key to living or dying: where women died needlessly, and in agony, because they could not afford to pay for surgery.

Women also died for other reasons. Anaemia was common and of 1200 women who gave birth in 1964, sixty-nine died during labour because blood transfusions were not available. I set up a blood bank, with the help of a peace corps volunteer who had been 'laid off' by the Eastern Nigerian Broadcasting Corporation after the coup which preceded the Biafran civil war. In the following six months only five women died. The figure was down to three in the next five months, but I had to leave the hospital. We had planned to move to Kenya, but with the outbreak of the Biafran civil war, I was evacuated with the children to England. We later rejoined Mike in Kenya.

A Woman's Right to Choose

In my training as a doctor, I was taught that abortion was wrong. It should only be performed if the woman's life was threatened by the continuance of the pregnancy. The first time I questioned this teaching was as a medical student when I saw a married woman, in her thirties with three children, die slowly from renal failure. She had syringed her uterus in an attempt to abort herself because she felt she could not cope with another child.

Her husband visited her every night and the love between them was obvious. She seemed no different from many women I have seen in the gynaecological wards or having babies. She was an ordinary housewife who had taken this desperate measure on her own and had died in the attempt. Nobody discussed with me the reasons for her death. It was accepted in silence. The 'finality' of her action was ignored.

I moved on as a medical student, with this experience buried and half-forgotten, through finals and marriage, house jobs and three babies in just over three years, until in Enugu I saw four young women die from attempts to induce abortion with a 'native' medicine. In Kenya I decided to specialise in obstetrics and gynaecology, and during my eighteen months in Nairobi I saw the effects of septic abortions daily. Every night we had an abortion list which included at least ten women with incomplete abortions which we had to complete.

On one occasion I was told that there was no legal way we could terminate the pregnancy of a young girl, only just eleven. She later returned to us, having had an illegal abortion, with a severe infection of the womb. I felt I should not have allowed this to happen. But I could see no way to perform an abortion. I did not know how; and if I had known, I did not know where I could have carried it out.

The questions which now began to worry me were: how could we as doctors refuse to help women who did not want to be pregnant? Was it ethical to refuse this help when the woman's only alternative was dangerous and unskilled assistance? Why did some of my medical colleagues – trained in Britain, members of the Royal College of Obstetricians and Gynaecologists (RCOG), and subscribing to the British medical code – lie to me about their illegal abortion activities, and appear to forget medical ethics when money was involved?

When, having returned to England in 1969, I had passed my exam for membership of the RCOG, the first step towards a consultant post, I decided to do some work in areas which I felt were neglected in orthodox NHS training. I studied family planning and venereal disease, and took psychosexual training. During this time I worked for a year with the Pregnancy Advisory Service, for the first month as a counselling doctor, and then as a gynaecologist, both seeing women before the operation and operating on them.

In these twelve months, there were only two women (out of 750) whose decision to request an abortion I felt to be wrong. I spent a long time advising both of them about a way round their problems. In both cases I delayed the operation for a week to give them time to reconsider. But both returned unconvinced and the abortions were carried out.

From the experience of talking to these 750 women, I learnt that it was impossible to pick out those who were so desperate that they would go anywhere to get an abortion from those who, given different laws, would accept the pregnancy. You had no choice but to believe what the woman told you as the doctor.

I learnt that some women have to know whether they *can* have an abortion before they can fully grasp their situation and be quite sure that is what they want. I quite quickly learnt to recognise those women who were ambivalent and needed more time to decide. And I learnt to spot those who were being pressured by their parents or partners into an unwanted abortion.

To me, the death of even one woman by illegal means, who could have had a legal safe abortion, is an unnecessary tragedy. But all doctors reach their positions on abortion by a different route. They all have their view of the gestational stage where they *feel* that the rights of the fetus take precedence over the mother's. Where that limit should be will continue to be debated hotly, but I would not like the law to be changed because it is now possible to keep alive a fetus of twenty-six weeks if superlative neonatal intensive care is available. I have interpreted 'viability' as natural viability, and I am still prepared, if really necessary, to do an abortion at twenty-six weeks. Very occasionally there are cases where women, usually young teenagers, do not reach the gynaecologist until over twenty-four weeks, the time limit that the DHSS have made the abortion charities accept 'voluntarily', and which most doctors would accept today. But I believe that it is the mother's view that should count. I have learnt from bitter experience that women will take the law into their own hands.

I can understand that people who have not seen women die from self-induced abortion may find it difficult to understand my own view. But such tragedies were not rare in England before the 1967 Abortion Act, although they were not as common as in Africa. Today the wards are no longer filled with women with infected abortions, and it is now rare to have women coming in with the haemorrhage once associated with 'spontaneous' abortion.

Doctors need to accept that ultimately the woman *does* make her decision, whatever the law says, and whatever her doctors think.

In July 1973, now a divorced mother of four, I took my young family to Gisborne, New Zealand. My post, newly created, was as a specialist in obstetrics, gynaecology, venereology and family planning. In Gisborne I found a 30 per cent extra-nuptial pregnancy rate and virtually no family planning service.

The abortion law was restrictive – much the same as in England prior to the 1967 Act – but, with the support of a progressive medical superintendent and a consultant psychiatrist, we established an abortion service. We also set up open-access family planning and venereology clinics and a regular review of the maternity service (80 per cent of women were looked after by their GPs and hospital midwives). During my three years in Gisborne, the perinatal mortality rate fell from twenty-nine per thousand deliveries to ten.

· CHAPTER 3 ·

Return to the London

The London Hospital, Mile End

Signs outside warn 'beware of falling masonry'. This is a small, very friendly, but old and tatty hospital. Though externally a 'dump', it is surprisingly progressive. Caring, considerate staff who treat women as individuals with minds of their own, although there are variations in practice and attitudes between different consultants ... student midwives and medical students present at the birth 'are not obtrusive'.

The New Good Birth Guide, 1983

Although my ideas were changing during my years abroad, it was not until working as a locum senior registrar at the West London Hospital, in 1976, shortly after my return to England, that I seriously reconsidered the conventional approach I had absorbed – and taught.

Watching a woman labouring to give birth to her first child, I thought that she needed some pain relief, and when she questioned my advice, I said, 'I've seen far more women in labour than you have.' The next day she told me that I had been quite wrong: she had felt she was doing well and the pethidine injection – and my dismissive advice – had upset her inner feelings and rhythm even though she had had a normal delivery. I realised that my interference had nearly ruined her feelings about the birth; I had interfered with her perceptions, marred her achievement.

I remembered this incident when, six months later, in November 1976, I went to work at Mile End Hospital as locum lecturer/honorary senior registrar to Professor Peter Huntingford. On our first visit to the labour ward we saw a woman pushing ineffectively in the second stage of labour. Outside I asked Peter why she had not been offered a forceps delivery which I thought she needed. He replied, 'Why interfere? The baby is all right, so is she. She is not ready to give up yet.'

These two experiences finally made me change my approach to childbirth. I was lucky to find myself working with Peter Huntingford at this relatively late stage in my career. His attitudes towards

18

women, combined with his intelligently informed experience, made him an excellent teacher.

Peter had had a brilliant academic career. He had been an editor of the *British Journal of Obstetrics and Gynaecology* and a professor at the early age of thirty-four. As clinical professor, he was based at the London. He had done a lot of research and was convinced that obstetric care in this country was going the wrong way. He felt that the rate of technological intervention was increasing too fast, without proper research to show whether it was actually improving birth for either the baby or the mother; and that doctors should be more sensitive in their attitude to women, involving them in a partnership where decisions were jointly made after the woman had been given the fullest information. He also thought that students, if they were to make worthwhile doctors, needed to observe good practice in action.

Peter took the chair on condition that his priority would not be academic research, but to establish a first-class service for women in Tower Hamlets.

Tower Hamlets was the name given in the 1960s to the new borough created out of the East End districts of Whitechapel, Bethnal Green, Stepney, Bow, Spitalfields, Poplar, Wapping and the Isle of Dogs. It is one of the most deprived areas in the country. Half of all households live below the official poverty line established by the Diamond Royal Commission in 1982, and the borough has the highest proportion of council housing in London. Of the sixteen districts covered by the North East Thames Regional Health Authority, Tower Hamlets has the highest proportion of single old people, of children in care, the highest rate of tuberculosis and of infant mortality.

In 1976, Peter moved the academic department away from the Whitechapel branch of the London Hospital and the Medical College to its less prestigious branch, the Mile End Hospital, because he hoped that with the proposed merger of Bart's, the London, and Queen Mary College, 'a major clinical academic presence at Mile End would be useful'. He set up an obstetric and gynaecological service where women were offered choice and treated as intelligent, thinking people. Although I had been a consultant for three years by now and was used to teaching, Peter's extensive theoretical and practical experience made ward rounds and seminar sessions fascinating.

I had always tried to inform people clearly so that they could make proper choices about their lives. But I learnt from Peter to cut out the unnecessary adjectives – 'just a *small* cut', 'only a *tiny* prick' – which at best confuse people, and at worst, as they reel from the unpleasantness of a painful penicillin injection, destroy their trust in the doctor.

During my medical training at the London Hospital in the fifties, the gynaecology clinic at Whitechapel had made a deep impression on me. It seemed to embrace everything that was wrong about the way women were treated by the health service. The women sat in skimpy gowns, on rows of hard seats only a couple of feet from examination cubicles in which incomplete plywood partitions were closed front and back by curtains. There was no privacy – a doctor commonly walked through, whisking aside the curtain to see who was lying on the bed, or not drawing the curtains fully before examining a woman. The voices of the doctors asking the most intimate questions could be heard clearly by those waiting their turn, but I doubt if any of the doctors wondered why the women whispered their replies.

It was the archetypal cattlemarket. No wonder students hated gynae – we 'clerked' women (took their medical histories) in an outer corridor, writing on boards projecting from the wall, with another group of women only a few feet away. It was pure chance if the registrar called you to see the same woman you had clerked, and there were so many patients that teaching was a very hit-and-miss affair.

When I returned to the London Hospital twenty years later, the only change which had taken place in that clinic was that students taking histories for patients were separated by small perspex screens. I quite understood why Peter Huntingford had moved to the Mile End site where the consulting rooms, though old, were at least solidly built, had changing cubicles and enabled women to speak about their problems without fear of being overheard.

In August 1977, when I was appointed senior lecturer, Peter put me in overall charge of all student teaching. At Mile End, we had organised the clinics so that a woman who agreed to being seen by a student had her history taken in a private room and was present, fully dressed, to comment on the student's interpretation of what she had said when the history was presented to the consultant. The student then examined the woman with a consultant or registrar.

At the end of each two month attachment I gave the students a questionnaire about the course. Consistently they said they preferred the experience gained in the Mile End clinic.

In the gynaecological clinics, I found that many of our patients came from the same kind of community as they had twenty years earlier – large, extended families, not given to complaining despite the adversity they often faced. Women often saw their mothers and sisters every day; family life, birth and death were very important. They appreciated the 'local' service we provided, which tried to meet the needs of the community.

There had been some changes in the local area during my years abroad and which I saw in the antenatal clinics: among the newer residents were Cypriot, West Indian, Somali, and Chinese families; Vietnamese 'boat people'; Sikhs from the Punjab; and Gujeratis from East Africa. But their numbers were small compared with the large community of Bengalis from Sylhet in Bangladesh. By 1985 the Bengali population accounted for almost half the births annually in Tower Hamlets. Although the paediatricians, supported by the obstetricians and a community physician, managed to get two interpreter posts funded by 1981, this was insufficient for our needs, and we had to continue to use husbands as interpreters which in obstetrics and gynaecology has considerable limitations.

Only a few women were so deeply religious that they would rather die than see a male doctor. But we knew that all of them preferred to see a woman. This was difficult for us, as a department, to arrange. It often leads to a heavy workload for women doctors, but it is a pressure which is hard to resist.

The Day Care Abortion Service

In 1977 Peter Huntingford won his battle to get funds to start a day care abortion service at Mile End, using the outpatient department. Partly as a result of his research into fetal monitoring, Peter had been a founder member of the anti-abortion organisation, the Society for the Protection of the Unborn Child. But he had completely changed his mind on the issue as he listened to women seeking abortion after the law was changed in 1967. Through our different backgrounds we both realised that the only person who could make the abortion decision was the woman herself. We felt that the service was crucial to the women of Tower Hamlets; that it was quite wrong that these women, from one of the poorest districts in the country, should have to pay for an abortion or continue with a pregnancy which they *knew* they could not cope with, physically, emotionally or financially.

Using non-medical counsellors, we provided an out-patient abortion service to women who were healthy and less than thirteen weeks pregnant. As the service became known to local GPs they began to refer all their patients who needed abortions to us. Cheap to run, the day care service at Mile End dealt with half the women needing abortions in the District as outpatients, and most of the rest were operated on as day cases in the ward.

Although the day care service freed gynaecological beds at Whitechapel, which should have shortened the waiting lists there, our colleagues were not altogether happy with the service. When I was suspended, Jean Richards told me that some of my colleagues' opposition towards me stemmed from the day care abortion service which 'had turned Tower Hamlets into the abortion capital of London'. In 1983, Jean Richards commissioned a study of the clients of our service for the District Health Authority. It remained 'confidential' and was never presented to the Health Authority – perhaps because it did not bear out the accusations that women from outside the borough were being accepted, nor the rumour that we were doing more late abortions than before. In fact, in 1983 only 3 per cent of women were more than seventeen weeks pregnant when they had abortions at the London, compared with 9 per cent in 1975.

Choice in Childbirth

We tried to offer women a choice of services in childbirth by sharing antenatal care with GPs who were interested in cooperating with us and by encouraging the midwives to regain their autonomy and take on home deliveries (providing telephone back-up during labour and hospital support if necessary). In 1975 Peter unsuccessfully tried to persuade the NHS consultants to allocate a few beds to GPs so that family doctors could have their own delivery unit in the London Hospital. He offered the GPs the use of his own beds at Mile End, and as an alternative, started a 'domino' ('domiciliary in-and-out') scheme where women with normal pregnancies are looked after by their own doctor and community midwives throughout the pregnancy and labour, and return home after only six hours in hospital.

GPs had the choice of seeing the woman throughout the pregnancy and labour or sharing the decision about the type of care with us. Naturally, if there were complications, they would refer the woman for a second opinion. What our colleagues appeared to dislike most is that we offered the GPs choice. They felt that the consultant should take the decision about the woman's delivery. Fundamentally, the issue was power.

In spite of his academic and clinical experience, Peter had found the position of professor difficult. The lack of funds to do the things necessary to upgrade the fabric of the department and set up a modern service contributed to the difficulty in creating a united department. And although Peter's hard work and dedication – both to the National Health Service and to the students – was not in doubt, there was unspoken animosity within the Division of Obstetrics and Gynaecology about the kind of services we were providing.

Peter gave up the Chair of Obstetrics and Gynaecology in 1981, moving to Maidstone to work as an NHS consultant. After he had left, a senior professor remarked that the only thing Peter gave the London Hospital was a 'certain dubious notoriety'. In retrospect, I see that he probably included me in the same category.

I was happy at Mile End, away from the medical politicking at Whitechapel, and I wanted to continue the work we had started in the Academic Unit. But my position was weakened by Peter's departure. A battle began in the Division of Obstetrics and Gynaecology where I was always outnumbered by four voices to one.

The Balance of Power Shifts

It was to be two years before the new professor took up his post and in the 'interregnum' many of the positive achievements brought about by Peter were quietly undermined and eroded. The balance of power and status began to shift back towards Whitechapel with the appointment of Trevor Beedham as consultant, previously one of our two senior registrars, in July 1981. Although Peter had written seven clinical and operating sessions at Mile End into the job description for this post, I found that after Trevor Beedham was appointed he was allowed to rewrite his timetable, transferring the major part of his input and half his workload to Whitechapel and joining their on-call rota.

I also found myself outmanoeuvred over the appointment of a locum senior lecturer, to tide us over the interim before a new professor took up his post. At less than twenty-four hours notice, I was summoned to an impromptu appointments committee of four – the then Dean of the London Hospital Medical College, Professor David Ritchie; the Chairman of the Academic Division of Surgery, Professor John Blandy; the Chairman of the Division of Obstetrics and Gynaecology, Leonard Easton (who was shortly to retire); and me, representing the Academic Unit of O and G.

Leonard Easton suggested that we promote our senior registrar to the locum post, and I proposed that the post be advertised, as we had seen some excellent candidates when interviewing Trevor Beedham, earlier in the year. As an example, I suggested that the Australian woman who had performed well at the earlier interview, had more experience than any of our senior registrars and was currently conducting a substantial research project, might respond to an advertised post.

After some discussion Professor Ritchie seemed to be in favour of advertising when Professor Blandy weighed in with a vote 'for the chap we know'. It was then that one of the panel mounted an amazing attack on the Australian woman, repeating gossip that she was a difficult woman to work with, continuing with innuendo about her personal life which it would be wrong to repeat. I was disgusted by this behaviour and so angry that I could hardly express my disapproval. I left the room abruptly.

I felt like handing in my resignation to protest at this method of filling a post, but a senior professor, Sidney Watkins, calmed me down. I was powerless; I had to accept the committee's decision to appoint the existing senior registrar as Peter's temporary replacement. But I knew that as a senior registrar, he would, at some stage, rely on the support of the other consultant obstetricians for promotion to a consultant post himself. Because of this he would be unlikely to support me in any discussion over the services to women in Tower Hamlets.

These two appointments were crucial to reducing the workload of the obstetric unit at Mile End Hospital. Instead, I found my workload increasing. After Peter left, GPs tended to send women with more difficult social and pyschological problems to me, and the referrals to the day care abortion unit rose to 1000 a year, nearly twice as many as our sessions allowed for. By 1982 I found that my share of the obstetric work at Mile End hospital had increased to the point where, even if we started at 8.30 a.m. and had a midwife do the bookings, I could no longer manage with one antenatal clinic a week.

Community Antenatal Care

For some time, I had been impressed by the work of Ken Boddy in Sighthill, and Ron Taylor and Luke Zander in Lambeth. They had extended the concept of 'shared care', the system of giving GPs some of the responsibility for women's antenatal care, to completely community-based schemes where women did not have to visit the hospital at all, even if they suffered from high-risk conditions like diabetes.

In the sixties and early seventies, antenatal care was almost entirely hospital-based. Women began to object that they were being treated like cattle, block-booked into impersonal hospital antenatal care units where there was nowhere for their children to play, and where they had to wait for hours to see a different doctor each time. The doctor they saw was often hurried and harassed, didn't explain things to them properly and they felt treated them as a walking incubator. The lack of continuity of care from both doctors and nurses in the hospital clinic could lead to missed test results, forgotten prescriptions, confusing advice, and lack of encouragement to ask questions.

Ken Boddy pioneered a community obstetric scheme at Sighthill Health Centre, on a housing estate in Edinburgh, in 1978. Luke Zander, Senior Lecturer in General Practice, and Professor Ronald Taylor, both of St Thomas's Hospital in Lambeth, extended this scheme so that in their area a hospital consultant visits local practices weekly to advise GPs and carry out joint consultations with patients.

After visiting their practice, I thought the best solution to the increased workload at Mile End was to hold such antenatal clinics in GPs' surgeries, involving the family doctors and community midwives in sharing the care. I was already meeting regularly with some of the newer, younger, vocationally trained GPs who were replacing the older family doctors, and in September 1982 I started the scheme with three group practices. I enjoyed the more informal contact with the women, got to know more of the community midwives and, as the GPs took on community obstetric care, began to meet with the midwives every Monday morning to make sure they had the advice and support they needed. This move increased the proportion of women I saw personally, and enabled the GPs to develop their obstetric skills.

I mentioned the scheme to my colleagues, who expressed neither interest nor disapproval. It was not until 1985, after a district report on perinatal mortality had commended this initiative, that Professor Grudzinskas, who had never before discussed the overall scheme with me, attacked my participation in it in front of my colleagues, two of whom nodded in agreement with him. In their view, it was a 'misuse of medical college funds' for a teaching consultant like myself to make antenatal visits to GPs' surgeries.

Hospital divisions are supposed to work by consensus, and doctors have to be tolerant of each other's practice. However, there is always a struggle over the allocation of beds, junior staff and operating sessions, which seems to me to be about power and status rather than how to provide the best patient care or student teaching. I was interested in providing a good service for the women and jointly planning how to do this in a deprived, working-class district with shrinking resources. When I found that the booking system of my colleagues at Whitechapel apparently favoured middle-class women from outside the area, I was frustrated when they refused to consider ideas for reworking the system or to examine data which would tell us how many of these women needed the specialised services of a teaching hospital.

In the summer of 1981 I talked with Professor Kass, with whom I had worked nearly twenty years earlier in Boston, telling him of the problems facing the department and the difficulty in getting unity and a sense of direction within the division. Senior registrar accreditation had been withdrawn by the RCOG – a vote of no-confidence in our training programme which damaged recruitment at both senior and junior registrar level just as we lost the experience and dedication of Peter Huntingford.

Professor Kass's advice was simple: 'Keep your head down, your mouth shut and get on with the work. Don't waste time in arguments but use data to make your points.' I took his advice. I worked hard with the students, enjoying the challenge of organising the final examinations, and was pleased and relieved when the students did well. I was left alone at Mile End and rarely saw my colleagues, except at the increasingly lengthy and acrimonious meetings of the Division of Obstetrics and Gynaecology, where even relatively minor and uncontentious matters about the delivery of care to women in Tower Hamlets seemed to take increasingly more time to resolve.

The Attack on the Day Care Abortion Service

The position of Chair of the Division of Obstetrics and Gynaecology rotates, by election, among the five consultants in the division. In November 1982, the chairman was John Hartgill. A New Zealander, John had been appointed as a consultant twenty-five years earlier, having trained at the London with Peter Huntingford. John looks younger than his sixty years and cultivates a charming 'I'm just a simple chap' manner.

While I was abroad on study leave that November, John circulated a document which had caused great argument in the division. He wrote that women over twelve weeks pregnant, or with medical problems (those in my opinion with most need of counselling), should go not to the day care abortion clinic where counselling was available, but directly to the consultants' gynaecology clinics, where there were no lay women counsellors and where many of our junior staff, as in other units, had a conscientious objection to abortion.

Fortunately he added a paragraph which said that GPs and women could choose their own consultant, so the GPs continued to refer to me and the circular made no difference to the working of the day care unit. Before Peter left he had warned me that John had opposed my re-appointment as senior lecturer in 1980, and although by 1982 John's dislike was apparent, I thought this was due to philosophical and practical differences in our approach to obstetrics and gynaecology, rather than to any personal antagonism or doubts about my competence.

The New Professor Arrives

By January 1983 we had a new professor. The Chair of Obstetrics and Gynaecology at the London Hospital and St Bartholomew's Medical Colleges had finally been advertised in the spring of 1982, nearly a year after Peter Huntingford left. I applied, somewhat unrealistically, as I knew that having had a female career pathway – juggling children, jobs and several moves to different countries – my CV was not that of the successful academic. I was not shortlisted, but, in conversation with the dean, David Ritchie, I expressed my view that we needed someone with the experience to deal with the conflict within the division.

The dean did not tell me who the candidates were. Nor did anyone else. It seemed extraordinary to me then – and still does – that the applicants were spirited round Mile End Hospital without meeting me and yet I would be the person to work most closely with the new professor. I was completely excluded from the appointment, and only learned who the candidates were because a registrar told me, having heard one of my consultant colleagues discuss them with his anaesthetist during an operation.

The appointments committee included, on the NHS side, John Hartgill, as Chairman of the Division, and Gordon Bourne, representing our sister hospital, Bart's, with whom we shared the joint professorship. Professor Ritchie and Professor Blandy represented the Medical College, while Professor Tim Chard represented St Bartholomew's Medical School. There were two university external assessors.

There were four older and more experienced candidates but the committee chose a relatively young man, who had got his MD in Professor Chard's department and worked for Gordon Bourne at Bart's. Gedis Grudzinskas was then thirty-eight years old. My initial impression was favourable. I remembered him as the only lecturer from Bart's who turned up to teach students without having to be reminded several times about the commitment. His research into placental proteins was laboratory-based – something we lacked. A fellow lecturer told me that he was a good politician. He had left Bart's and returned to Sydney as Senior Lecturer at the North Shore Hospital eighteen months earlier. In the summer of 1982, before he took up his appointment, he came over to England to visit the department. Over dinner he seemed friendly and enthusiastic. I met him again in October, when, although the dean had recommended me as the college representative on an appointments committee for a consultant post (Mr Easton's replacement), my consultant colleagues objected to my participation and insisted that Gedis Grudzinskas was brought over from Australia. During this visit I introduced him to all the staff at Mile End Hospital and sought his advice on how to respond to the attack on the day care abortion service. Over the next two months we had several telephone conversations, and when he took up his appointment in January 1983, I was hopeful that his pure science interests and my psychosocially orientated research would complement each other to produce a well-rounded academic department.

Different Approaches

During the first year of his appointment Gedis and I had several discussions about improving teaching for the students and training for the registrars. There were already indications that our clinical approach was very different. On two occasions Gedis expressed 'concern' about my clinical practice. The first time, he seemed worried about the use of prostaglandin pessaries for induction, which he called a 'research procedure'. I was puzzled by his use of the term 'research procedure' and quoted some published papers about the use of prostaglandins with which he appeared to be unfamiliar. The second time, the issue was abortion – he was unhappy about my decision to terminate the advanced pregnancy of a twelve-year-old girl. She had been referred to me by her GP when already twenty-five weeks pregnant. Recent improvements in intensive neonatal care mean that it is just possible for babies of this gestational age to survive. However, without such technology their lungs are too immature to support life, and in my opinion this child was too young to continue with the pregnancy, cope with a baby, or go through the trauma of giving a baby up for adoption.

So without delay I arranged to start her 'labour', using an epidural to relieve pain. During our conversation about this, Gedis told me he needed a summary of the case so that he could protect me from the criticism of my NHS colleagues. At the time, I believed him.

As an academic and senior lecturer in the professorial department, I was answerable to the professor for my research and teaching. However, as holder of an honorary NHS consultant contract (I was paid by the college but worked for the Health District), I was a consultant in my own right and neither the professor, nor any other doctor, could direct my clinical decisions as long as they were within the bounds of acceptable medical practice. I was, therefore, surprised by this interference from a man who, although my senior in the academic hierarchy, had considerably less clinical experience than I did. I thought his behaviour could perhaps be attributed to a lack of administrative experience and initial difficulties in managing the delicate balance between the NHS input into the division and our academic unit. It was not until December, at the end of Gedis' first year, that hopes of a creative and friendly working partnership were dashed completely.

The First Major Dispute

The first substantial point of conflict concerned our response to the District Strategic Plan, which forecast less money and fewer beds for Tower Hamlets. We discussed the issue within the Division of Obstetrics and Gynaecology, where John Hartgill (then the Chairman) and Gedis Grudzinskas drew up a plan which meant losing twenty beds, two operating sessions and two junior staff, in order to achieve centralisation on the Whitechapel site. At the October division we reached a compromise but the following day, without consulting me first, they presented a changed plan to the District Administrator leaving out the safeguards I had negotiated and in addition cutting another ten beds. In the November division I expressed my disapproval of their action (i.e. changing our agreed position without consultation) but reiterated my support for centralisation of services. However when the plan was presented to the District Health Authority in December, by John and Gedis, the way the case was made deeply concerned me. I told the Professor that I thought the plan could lead to an inadequate service for the women of Tower Hamlets and that the option of centralisation on the Mile End site had not been adequately costed or considered. I could no longer keep silent.

The professor ordered me not to make a move that was contrary to the division's plan. I reminded him that, as this was a National Health Service rather than an academic matter, he could not direct my actions. It seemed to me there were two options. Either I went secretly to the District Health Authority members and told them my anxieties, pointing out how the case presented to them had been poorly researched and costed and, in my view, distorted to make the case which suited my colleagues; or I could use the medical advisory system to present a paper arguing my own position. I decided that the second way was the more honest, and I duly wrote a paper which included perinatal and maternal mortality figures to counter allegations the professor had made that obstetrics at Mile End was not safe. I addressed the paper to the Final Medical Committee, the body which is composed of the Chairs of all the Divisions in the hospital, and concerns itself with questions of policy, staffing and the provision of services. It also puts forward the consensus view of all the consultants about matters of district policy, via a representative on the District Health Authority. My paper was, however, not discussed, and they agreed to support the division's plan.

The Division of Obstetrics and Gynaecology passed a motion censuring my action in presenting my dissenting paper to the Final Medical Committee. They referred this motion to the FMC who declined to discuss the matter further. But later its chairman, Professor Sidney Watkins, remarked to me, 'It seems to be a crime to express a contrary opinion in the Division of O and G.'

I then received a letter from the professor:

20 February 1984. Professor Gedis Grudzinskas to Wendy Savage:

Further to our discussion on 12 January 1984 and 17 February 1984, I wish to confirm that, having considered at length your activities as senior lecturer since my appointment over twelve months ago, I am concerned about their counterproductive nature, which is detrimental to your position and the interests of the Academic Unit and the Medical College.

Despite repeated verbal warnings, you continue to fail to coordinate your activities with those of your colleagues in the Academic Unit, and the College and Hospital Divisions.

As head of your department, I have, over the past year, and after many discussions with you and our other colleagues in the Hospital Division, secured agreements which should allow us to offer better clinical service as well as to improve the standard of teaching and research. To deliberately, and in my absence, take active steps to undermine these agreed plans (to which you were a party) is unacceptable to me as head of your department. In addition you have refrained repeatedly from acting in accordance with directions aimed at the rational deployment of the Academic Unit resources for the purposes of enhancing our teaching and research potential within the context of our clinical service commitments, conducted jointly with our NHS colleagues. This behaviour is not only disloyal to me personally, and to your colleagues, but it has compromised your position in the Academic Unit, the College and Divisions, at a critical time in the history of this unit.

These matters are raised in detail with you formally, in order to emphasise the seriousness with which I view this subject. From a senior member of the unit, I consider that respect for the position held, loyalty to the Head of the Unit, action in accordance with the head's directions on teaching and research, and the relationship of the Unit to our NHS colleagues are reasonable expectations.

It is of prime importance that you consider your responsibilities to the aspirations and agreed strategy of the unit a major priority. Furthermore, if you continue to act in this inappropriate manner without any significant change in your activities, I shall be forced to advise the review of your own employment positions. It is only fair to warn you that in these circumstances this may lead to termination of your employment.

The professor had sent copies of this letter to Professor Mike Floyer, the new Dean of the Medical College, Professor John Blandy, Chairman of the Academic Division of Surgery, and Professor Tim Chard, who represented St Bartholomew's Hospital on the Academic Unit.

Shocked by this turn of events, I went to see the professor in his office. At our meeting, Professor Grudzinskas told me that I was not doing enough research (although I had two grants and three research assistants in post) and was doing too much clinical work. I agreed that I was doing more clinical work than the six sessions which my job description allocated to me, and I explained that I could cut this down if there was more input at Mile End from the senior registrar, who was increasingly spending most of his time at Whitechapel.

Giving me no specific example, the professor then said that

people were 'sniggering and laughing at me', that my colleagues did not like my clothes, my politics or my style, that I had harassed a lecturer, that my standing in the Division of O and G had fallen, and that I was 'disruptive'.

I went to see Mike Floyer, who was supportive and listened to my explanations about the dispute. He told me that he had reminded Professor Grudzinskas that without me the student teaching would have collapsed after Peter Huntingford had left. He offered to see us together, and I thanked him and said that perhaps we could sort it out between ourselves.

I thought it wise, as my job was at stake, to seek legal advice about the terms in which I should reply to the professor's letter.

5 March 1984. Wendy Savage to Professor Gedis Grudzinskas:

I appreciate the full and frank discussions that I have had with you and separately with the Dean, since receiving your letter of 20.2.84. These have clarified for me some of your anxieties about the Academic Unit and I hope I have reassured you that I have not been disloyal to you either personally or as head of the unit.

I was sorry that after the meeting we had on 2.3.84 you did not feel able to withdraw the letter, as I had asked you to, which leaves me no alternative but to reply to you in legalistic terms.

Your letter of the 20.2.84 purports to be a formal warning which may lead to temination of my employment. I must tell you that I reject totally your view that any such warning is justified, because your allegations in the first three paragraphs are untrue. In particular I have not undermined agreed plans but have merely exercised my right to express my opinion about those plans to the Final Medical Committee. In any case, I believe you have seriously overemphasised the impact that my representation had on hospital and college staff outside the Division of Obstetrics and Gynaecology.

I am able to state quite categorically that your allegations are untrue because I know that I have fulfilled my job description to the best of my ability. It is significant that you have not in your letter given any details of a single occasion when I have failed to carry out any proper direction or have failed to co-ordinate my activities with those of my colleagues. You claim to have raised matters in detail in your letter, but have not done so. If you have any specific complaints, please let me know what they are so that I may have the opportunity to revise them.

However, I hope that, avoiding further recriminations about the past, we as members of the Academic Unit can sit down with the other members of the Division of Obstetrics and Gynaecology and jointly find a way forward. As no individual acting alone can be expected to heal the wounds that have been incurred in the past, I wonder if the help of some arbitrator or negotiating body should be sought? If all five of us could sit down and together resolve some of the deep-seated, but unexpressed differences which divide us, perhaps with the help of the 'Three Wise Persons' or someone from outside the London Hospital, we could reconcile our viewpoints and find a way of working productively in the future.

Within the Medical College, might not the problems associated with both of us having too much to do, be solved by asking the District Health Authority to pay for enough of our sessions to fund another Senior Lecturer, perhaps with a more research orientated role to strengthen our small department?

As I said to you on 17.2.84 I remain confident that together we can build a good department, and whatever the difficulties that have occurred in the past year I will support and have supported you in that aim.

My reference to the 'Three Wise Persons' was to the special professional panel, colloquially known as the 'Three Wise Men' to whom doctors can in confidence refer colleagues whose behaviour, they consider, because of illness, drug or alcohol abuse, is putting patients at risk. I had briefly discussed this possibility with the Professor of Psychiatry, who was a member of the panel, and he thought they could be used in the way I suggested.

The professor briefly acknowledged this letter on the seventh of March, together with his arrangements for 'cover' during his leave. They did not include me, in spite of my official responsibility to deputise clinically and academically for the professor in his absence. On his return from holiday he wrote to me again:

19 March 1984. Professor Gedis Grudzinskas to Wendy Savage:

Thank you for your letter of the 5 March 1984 which, in addition to other matters, requests clarification of my expectations of the Senior Lecturer position outlined in my letter of 2 February 1984. From your reply it seems that you have not fully understood or appreciated the points I raised in relation to your role and responsibilities as a senior member of the department.

As you are aware, it is the duty of the academic clinical staff at all levels to undertake teaching and research, in addition to clinical service duties under the direction of the Head of Department. My expectations are, therefore, firstly that you conduct your clinical service duties within the six clinical sessions stated in your contract; secondly that you participate in other clinical activities only if the major implications of your involvement are teaching and research.

Proposed involvement in such extra clinical duties is to be approved by the Head of Department, and finally to promote by teaching, supervision and research, the advancement of obstetrics and gynaecology in the remaining five sessions.

. . . The issue is your failure to comply with my directions and the agreed plans of the division. In these circumstances it would not be appropriate to involve a third party. It is important therefore that I refer you back to my original letter of 20 February 1984 and reiterate that you consider your responsibilities to the aspirations and agreed strategy of the division as your first priority.

6 April 1984. Wendy Savage to Professor Gedis Grudzinskas:

Thank you for your letter of 19 March 1984. It is perfectly true that I did not understand the points that you raised in your letter of 20.2.84. That is why I asked you for clarification but your latest letter does not provide this. You have given no instance in which I have failed to comply with the duties set out in my job description and I do not find your statement of your expectations helpful, because it is almost entirely negative: apart from reminding me of my obligation to conduct six clinical sessions and five teaching and research sessions, you merely tell me that I must not participate in other clinical activities without your approval. Could you please tell me what you wish me to do. I will then do my best to fulfil your proper and reasonable expectations. I would like to repeat that I cannot accept that my expressions of opinion on the District Strategic Plan are in conflict with the duties of my position or can be properly restrained by your directions. This view has been confirmed by legal advice. I would ask you to read again my letter of 6 March, 1984, which was written in a spirit of friendship and in the hope that we can build an active, modern department of obstetrics and gynaecology.

18 May 1984. Professor Gedis Grudzinskas to Wendy Savage:

I have considered at length your letter of 6 April 1984. I must conclude from your correspondence that you have demonstrated a lack of insight into the problems I have raised in my letters, and the manner in which I should like you to deal with them. I would, therefore, like to terminate this correspondence.

I believe that the contents of my letters have been quite explicit concerning my requirements of a senior member of this department, and I shall review your performance over the next few months to determine whether there has been compliance with my directions. If this turns out not to be the case, I shall be forced once again to raise the subject of termination of your employment.

29 May 1984. Wendy Savage to Gedis Grudzinskas:

Your letter of the 18 May 1984 leaves me no alternative but to ask the dean to meet with us on his return from holiday, so that you can tell me in his presence, in what way you consider that I am failing in my duties, so that I know what to do to meet your wishes.

I must make it clear once again that you have not specified hitherto where you consider me at fault: clearly I cannot take any steps to resolve the situation until I know this.

The professor refused the three-way meeting I had asked for, and the issue of my protest at the way the plans had been put before the District Health Authority was not discussed again. But although I did not know it, the professor had already taken steps to secure an investigation into my clinical practice, which led to my suspension in April 1985.

· CHAPTER 4 ·
The Hidden Agenda

In April 1984, a young Bangladeshi woman, Mrs U, had her second baby at the London Hospital (Mile End) under my care. Her first baby had been delivered by Caesarean section, and now this second baby had turned late in the pregnancy to a breech position (bottom first).

It seemed likely that she would need a Caesarean again, but I decided to allow her a 'trial of labour' first. I have come to understand that it is important for some women to feel that they have tried to deliver a baby vaginally even if, at the end of the trial of labour, they end up having a Caesarean section. Ten years ago I would not have understood that, and would have thought that there was no point in a woman labouring in vain. I have learnt since then that some women need to know, through their own bodies, that the baby is not going to deliver vaginally.

When Mrs U was transferred to the labour ward, the duty registrar, Toby Fay, confirmed with her and her husband that they wanted to try a normal labour, even though the baby was in the breech position.

In a normal, straightforward delivery, the birth is handled entirely by the midwives. In the case of a delivery which may be complicated by, for example, a breech presentation, the duty registrar will oversee the birth, following a plan of management laid down for this labour by the consultant. If anything arises during the labour which this registrar cannot deal with, he or she contacts the consultant to confer, seek approval or confirm changes in the plan for delivery. If a labour is not straightforward, I like the registrar to keep in touch with me throughout; this differs from the practice of some consultants, who lay down a set of 'protocols' for the members of their team to refer to. But I believe it allows for more flexibility to manage each woman's labour individually, and is a better way of helping junior staff to develop their skills.

Because Dr Fay was due to take his membership examination for the Royal College of Obstetricians and Gynaecologists, the MRCOG, we had discussed the ways in which my plan of management for Mrs U's delivery would differ from the 'textbook' management of this kind of case. I had explained to him the two reasons why I thought it important to let a woman feel some contractions if she wanted to, even though a Caesarean section was likely. The first was that women accepted the need for and the discomfort of a Caesarean section more easily if they had felt physically that they were going to be unable to deliver normally. The second was that if they were not convinced of its necessity, they might try and deliver at home the next time they became pregnant. In England with good roads and ambulances this was not as dangerous as in the Third World. My experience in Africa had shown me however (and there was always a possibility that the Us might return to Bangladesh) that there was a high risk of the mother and baby dying if the scarred uterus ruptured miles from the hospital.

Three successive registrars looked after Mrs U during her labour, which was not carried out exactly as I had planned. The baby, a boy, was eventually born by Caesarean section and was well at his birth. Unexpectedly, he became ill forty-eight hours later and, despite excellent and energetic treatment by the paediatricians, he died on 4 May, the following week.

I suggested to the baby's parents that if we did a post-mortem, it would enable us to find out exactly why their baby had died. They discussed it with their Imam, who said that it would be against their religion, and, respecting their wishes, a post-mortem was not carried out.

On Monday May 13, Trevor Beedham, now the new Chairman of the Division of Obstetrics and Gynaecology, came to tell me that Professor Grudzinskas had asked him to set up an investigation into my handling of Mrs U's delivery. I felt some sympathy for his obvious embarrassment at having to relay the professor's decision, but I was disturbed that he apparently did not know what kind of an enquiry the professor had in mind.

The paediatricians (doctors who specialise in the care of children) had suggested that the reason the baby had suddenly

become ill two days after his birth was because the delivery had
produced a tentorial tear, which is a split in the delicate membrane
between parts of the brain. If a baby's head is subjected to either a
lot of moulding (squashing the head out of shape in the bony
pelvis) or sudden changes of pressure (for example, if forceps are
used high in the pelvis, or if the baby's head passes very quickly
through the pelvis in a vaginal breech delivery), the tear may reach
a large blood vessel in this membrane and cause bleeding inside the
skull. This causes pressure on the brain and the baby usually dies
shortly after birth.

I was doubtful whether this had happened in this case. In my
experience, babies with this kind of bleeding were unwell from the
time they were born, although symptoms of pressure on the brain,
such as jitteriness and fits, or paleness due to loss of blood, might be
revealed as much as six or twelve hours later. This baby was not
unwell when he was born, and fed well for at least a day. I thought
it more likely that the intracranial bleeding (inside the skull) was a
result of the blood clotting problem which had also been diagnosed
when he became ill.

Although Mrs U's labour was not successful, Hani Youssef, my
registrar, who had carried out the Caesarean, had told me that the
delivery of the baby was uneventful. I told Trevor that there was no
evidence in the case notes to suggest that my registrar had
delivered the baby badly, producing a tentorial tear, and I did not
think that the baby's death was due to the labour or delivery.

As we parted I remarked that I thought that whatever worries
the professor had about this delivery would be answered by a full
discussion at the perinatal mortality meeting, which was due to
review the U case the following day.

Tuesday, 14 May 1984

I arrived at Whitechapel before 8 a.m., slightly earlier than usual,
to see a young woman whose heart had stopped in the anaesthetic
room the previous Saturday. Despite the doctors taking the correct
action immediately she had suffered severe brain damage, and it
was already clear to me that there was no hope when I saw her and
her family on Sunday. This morning her condition was unchanged
and the nurses told me that test results for brain death would be
ready after my gynae clinic and teaching session. I spoke to the
woman's mother and husband briefly, arranging the harrowing

interview for the afternoon when the results would be known.

It took place in the hostel where relatives stay when patients are very ill or live far away: a dark and gloomy place, in spite of attempts to cheer it up with bright curtains and modern furniture. On this day the small room was crowded, silent and filled with cigarette smoke. I broke the news as gently as I could.

It was 5.15 p.m. when I left the family for the perinatal mortality meeting where Mrs U's case was to be discussed. I hurried through the hospital garden, deeply saddened by this tragedy – a young woman, suffering a cardiac arrest while her first pregnancy miscarried. I did not feel like arguing when Trevor, who was waiting outside the lecture theatre where the meeting was to be held, told me that Mrs U's case would not be discussed. I thought we would discuss it the following month. It did not cross my mind that Professor Grudzinskas would then postpone the case discussion for the June, July and August meetings.

Although I did not know it, Trevor had already acquired and summarised the case notes of Mrs U and discussed the matter with Sotiris Argyrou, the District Administrator, Professor Watkins, the Chairman of the Medical Council, and the Medical Protection Society.

Nearly two years later, Trevor Beedham told the enquiry panel that he had been advised by the Medical Protection Society not to discuss the case at the perinatal mortality meeting; to consider the implications of pursuing an enquiry; and to follow his conscience. However, it emerged that this was only part of the advice given to him. When Professor Watkins, whom he had also consulted, learned of Trevor's evidence to the enquiry, he wrote a letter to my solicitor, a copy of which was sent to the enquiry chairman.

6 March 1986. Professor Sidney Watkins to Brian Raymond:

. . . Mr Beedham and I agree, that the content of the discussion in question (May 1984) went as follows: . . . [I] said to him that it was extremely difficult ever to prove incompetence. I read to him the requirements, quoted in a legal case in which I had been involved, that have to be established as facts to prove an allegation of deviation from normal practice. At this stage I said that if I was in his position I would have nothing to do with an enquiry, 'I wouldn't touch it with a barge pole.' My final statement was that, 'I would not wish to see the lid taken off the Pandora's box of incompetence, as the effects would be widespread and damaging and one could not predict where the damage would stop.'

In spite of Professor Watkins' advice, the move for an enquiry pressed ahead. Trevor, in his capacity as Chairman of the Division of Obstetrics and Gynaecology, circulated a letter to my colleagues and administrators which, while passing the ball back to Professor Grudzinskas' court, also served as the formal request for an enquiry to Sotiris Argyrou. (In fact Argyrou had already been informally consulted.) The letter was not marked private or confidential and fuelled gossip within the London Hospital and wider medical circles. It was tantamount to issuing a public statement that I was incompetent and not fit to be allowed near patients. However, as Trevor Beedham was to admit at the enquiry, many of the 'facts' within it were incorrect and misleading.

21 May 1984. Trevor Beedham to Professor Gedis Grudzinskas:

I have now had time to assess the request made by yourself, the Director of Midwifery, Mr Oram and Mr Hartgill for an enquiry into the management and delivery of Mrs A...U..., hospital number .... She was booked under the care of Mrs W. D. Savage, the Senior Lecturer, who personally supervised her.

When I discussed Mrs U with Mrs Savage on the 13th May 1984, she described her management as 'controversial' and thought it unlikely that anyone else in London would have managed that case in that way. She was not absolutely sure that Mrs U and her husband clearly understood the controversial aspects of her management and certainly there was no written agreement for a research procedure. During the course of the labour, and over some hours, whilst Mrs Savage continued to direct events personally, the duty medical staff became so fearful of the outcome that they telephoned Mr Oram, yourself and Mr Hartgill.

Since the discussion with Mrs Savage, I have taken further advice about Mrs U's care and have been told that further public discussion should be postponed. In consequence the case was not presented at the Perinatal Meeting on 14 May 1984.

I am concerned about the effects of such 'controversial' management (which is not a recognised research procedure) on our junior staff and midwives, and about their ability to maintain the best standards of patient care in such circumstances. The anxieties of the junior staff appear to be reflected by the consultants who support the request for an enquiry and who, for some time, have not been prepared to invite the Senior Lecturer to cross-cover for them. In view of the gravity of this problem, I think that initially the solution must be sought within the Academic Unit, but because of its wider implications I am sending copies of this letter to the

District Administrator, the Chairman of the Medical Council and the Secretary of Mile End Hospital.

It was only at the enquiry, one year and nine months later, that five damaging statements in this letter were publicly shown to be untrue:

Firstly, Trevor Beedham had stated that the call for an enquiry into my practice came from the Professor of Obstetrics, Gedis Grudzinskas, the Director of Midwifery, and my consultant colleagues, David Oram and John Hartgill. But the enquiry panel was later to examine a letter which the Director of Midwifery wrote to Trevor Beedham in June 1985, denying that she had asked for a special enquiry in the U case, David Oram was to tell the panel: 'I do not recall putting my hand up and initiating things'; and John Hartgill's written statement, prepared for the enquiry, was to be completely silent on this point.

Professor Grudzinskas, on the other hand, was to recall that he had asked for the initial inquiry into the U case, and that he spoke with Trevor Beedham in his capacity as Chairman of the Division of O and G. The impression created in the letter, however, was that all the other consultants and the midwives were united in their anxieties about my practice and its effect on patients.

Secondly, in his evidence to the enquiry, Trevor Beedham was to concede that I had not described my management of Mrs U's case as controversial. Nor, as he agreed under cross-examination, had I suggested that it was a 'research procedure'. This was a very damaging allegation, suggesting that I was experimenting on my patients without their knowledge or consent – using women as guinea pigs.

Thirdly, Trevor Beedham's letter claimed that over some hours during the course of the labour, duty medical staff became so fearful of the outcome that they telephoned David Oram, John Hartgill and the professor for advice. But the enquiry revealed that only one person had telephoned for advice, making two calls within one hour *before* labour commenced. Toby Fay, David Oram's registrar, telephoned David, and then the professor (but not John Hartgill) because he wanted advice on how he should react if he was asked to carry out a plan of management with which he disagreed.

Fourthly, the other consultants had never told me that they were

unhappy for me to cover for them during holidays or illness. David
Oram told the enquiry that he had no anxieties about my clinical
ability to cover his practice; the only reason he did not ask me to
cross-cover with him was that it was administratively easier to
share with Trevor Beedham, who worked, as he did, on both sites
whereas I worked almost exclusively at Mile End.

Soon after the professor's arrival in 1983, a new duty rota was
circulated in which one month I was covering at Mile End paired
with John Hartgill at Whitechapel, while for the other three
months the younger consultants were on call for both sites. When
I protested about this change, never discussed at the divisional
meeting, which could be seen as a lowering of my status, and
which I felt was an attempt to isolate me, the professor implied
that this was John Hartgill's idea, and that the situation would
be resolved when obstetrics was centralised. There was never, at
any time, an implication that there was any question about my
competence.

At this time Professor Watkins was in his third year as Chairman
of the Final Medical Committee and Medical Council. The paths
of obstetricians and neurosurgeons rarely cross, but in 1980 I had
referred a young woman dying of cervical cancer for treatment of
her intractable pain to Professor Watkins. Early the next year he
had referred me a patient who was twenty-nine weeks pregnant
when she was admitted unconscious with a brain tumour. I
advised against doing an elective Caesarean section prior to the
long operation he planned to remove her brain tumour. But
because of the risk of haemorrhage or raising the pressure in the
brain during the second stage of labour, Professor Watkins asked
me to do an elective Caesarean at forty weeks and she had a healthy
8lb baby who has done well.

During this time I got to know Sid Watkins – the only
person at the London who makes me laugh! When I got Trevor
Beedham's letter on 22 May 1984, I was extremely upset, and rang
Sid for advice. He asked if my visit was official or unofficial.
Somewhat startled, I replied 'official' because it was in his capacity
as Chairman of the Medical Council (see chapter 5, p. 63) that I
wanted his help. I told him what had happened in the U case,
and as a neurosurgeon he agreed that bleeding into the head was
more likely to happen following a blood-clotting disorder than the
other way round. He told me that Trevor Beedham, as Chairman

of the Division, had sought his advice formally and that he had told him to have nothing whatsoever to do with setting up an enquiry, and that he had also advised him that incompetence was almost impossible to prove.

Sid knew what problems I had faced in the Division of O and G and also had little expectation that the dean would support me. I had told him how inaccurate and damaging Trevor Beedham's letter was but when I went to see him he had not yet received his copy of the letter. It was not until August of 1985 that I learned that he had never received it. In retrospect that was very important in understanding why I was not more anxious. I knew that he met Sotiris Argyrou, the District Administrator, every week and assumed that Sid had given him the same advice as he had given to Trevor Beedham.

Thursday, 12 July 1984

Acting on the advice of Hempsons, the solicitors allocated to me by the Medical Defence Union, I complied with Professor Grudzinskas' requests for a report on the handling of Mrs U's case – despite the fact that he had no clinical (as opposed to academic) authority over me, and was not, strictly speaking, entitled to make such a request. I sent the report with a covering note, pointing out the inaccuracies in Trevor's letter. I wanted to circulate copies of this note because so many people had seen the letter, but Hempsons advised me 'not to send copies to anyone else for the time being'. With hindsight, I think this was an error. It allowed the secret manoeuvres to continue.

The proposed discussion of the U case was postponed once more at the June perinatal mortality meeting, and again in July, at Professor Grudzinskas' request.

I had promised Mr and Mrs U that I would have a full discussion of their child's death with them after the meeting. Because of the postponements I had to write to them in June, and again in July, to explain that it had not yet been discussed within the hospital.

Tuesday, 5 August 1984

After cancelling the perinatal mortality review for the *fourth* time, the professor talked over Mrs U's case with me when he called at my office to borrow my dictating machine. I asked if this was the formal discussion of the case which he had proposed, but he replied that it wasn't, as he didn't yet have the X-rays and the cardiotocographic (CTG) strips which are the recordings of the baby's heart beat. (They were found and sent to the professor in early October.)

I wrote again to Mr and Mrs U, explaining that their case would not be discussed at the August meeting either. Although I was not, at the time, aware of the reasons for the repeated postponement of the U perinatal mortality discussion, it was nonetheless a source of concern to me, because it denied the Us a proper, formal consideration of the circumstances surrounding the death of their baby and made them feel that the hospital, and its doctors, were not giving them a straightforward, honest explanation. If the normal discussion had taken place, however, it would have been necessary for Professor Grudzinskas and Trevor Beedham to inform me openly that the handling of the case was being taken up with the administrators. As it happened it was not until my suspension in April 1985 that I really knew what was going on.

In early July the Us consulted the Community Health Council. However, they did not at that time wish to press a formal complaint. They went back to the CHC in August, the CHC wrote to Mr Argyrou, who forwarded the letter to me. I arranged to meet them with the paediatrician who had cared for the baby on 24 September. It was at this meeting that I realised for the first time quite how the case had been presented to the parents. I told the Us that as there had been no post-mortem the cause of death could only be a 'guess' and that, even if it were true, which I doubted, that the baby had suffered a tentorial tear, then an earlier Caesarean section would have made no difference.

Since my explanation was accepted in front of the secretary of the Community Health Council who was advising the parents, and as this complaint had come through the District Administrator, I thought the matter was closed.

In addition, as I heard nothing further from the professor, I assumed my report to him had been satisfactory. After October, neither the professor, nor Trevor Beedham, nor any other person, spoke to me about Mrs U's case again, until after my suspension.

The formal action had actually begun in the summer of 1984 when, without my knowledge, the U case was considered by the district team of officers (the medical, nursing and administrative officers responsible for the running of the health service in each district).

The team of officers could have dealt with the matter in several ways: they could have considered the case report I had prepared for the professor; they could have used the obstetric databank – one of the most extensive in the country – to see whether there was any evidence of higher mortality or morbidity (death or complications) in my practice, to put this isolated case in context; in view of the conflict between me and my colleagues within the Division of Obstetrics and Gynaecology, they could have reasonably sought an informal, independent opinion. They could have sought the advice of the RCOG or discussed the situation with the Chairman of the Medical Council of the London Hospital. And they could have asked me for my views.

The team of officers did none of these things. Instead, they took an extraordinary step: they asked my two younger and less experienced colleagues, Trevor Beedham and Gedis Grudzinskas, the men who had originally asked for an enquiry into the case, to comment on my management and my fitness to carry out my duties.

At this stage the only evidence before the district team of officers that my conduct was questionable was that in the opinions of Professor Grudzinskas and Trevor Beedham this was so. But instead of seeking confirmation from others of the 764 consultant obstetricians in England and Wales, they returned to these two for further information.

Wednesday, 15 August 1984. Dr Jean Richards to Professor J. G. Grudzinskas/Trevor Beedham:

It was agreed to formally ask you to present two reports as follows:
1. A report on the particular incident involving the death of the baby. They need to know whether any departmental policies need to be reviewed in the light of this incident, etc. and the opinion on the clinical management of the case.
2. We need a report on the competence of the consultant concerned to carry on in clinical obstetric care. The initial reports we had from Mr Beedham indicated that there was considerable doubt on this matter. The authority needs to be assured that the clinician is safe to continue managing obstetric patients.

The first of these queries is standard management practice, but the second is most unusual. If competence is questioned, the Regional

Medical Officer usually seeks an independent opinion via the RCOG or their regional legal department, using doctors skilled in dealing with medical negligence claims.

Thursday, 20 September 1984. Trevor Beedham to Dr Jean Richards:

. . . My enquiries at the time indicated that the duty staff made every effort (including contacting three of my colleagues) to change the management which they regarded as having a predictably morbid outcome. Once these circumstances became known to me I was informally advised by my defence organisation (in a situation which they regarded as indefensible) to inform the officers of the Health Authority in the interests of patient care, and to refute complicity . . . I have been advised not to comment about the ability of the consultant concerned to carry on clinical obstetric care, thus I cannot give the Authority the assurance it seeks.

Trevor Beedham wrote his initial letter in May, some eight days after he had spoken to me, but by September when he replied to the formal request from the District Medical Officer to comment on my competence, he had had ample time to confirm whether his initial understanding of the situation was correct. His use of the privileged 'informal' advice given to him by the Medical Protection Society also strengthened the case against me.

A day earlier Professor Grudzinskas had also written to Dr Richards, sending a copy of his letter to the dean and Trevor Beedham.

Wednesday, 19 September 1984. Professor Gedis Grudzinskas to Dr Jean Richards:

I regret that I am unable to give the Authority the assurance that the clinician is safe to continue managing obstetric patients. Firstly, I have received legal advice that such a judgement should not be made by an immediate colleague such as myself, and secondly, I am currently enquiring into at least three additional obstetric and gynaecological incidents involving this consultant.

At the enquiry Trevor Beedham was to agree that he knew about and had seen this letter, although he couldn't recall the last sentence.

Tuesday, 27 September 1984
I knew nothing of the new investigation into 'at least three additional cases', but there was an indication that the informal

enquiry into the U case was continuing. Dr Jean Richards mentioned to me on the telephone that she was looking for the case notes as she was thinking of sending them to Gordon Bourne, the Regional Assessor, because the Division of Obstetrics and Gynaecology had asked her to set up an enquiry under the terms of DHSS circular HM (61)112.

I had never heard of HM (61)112, but I remember responding sharply to the suggestion that the Division of Obstetrics and Gynaecology had asked for an enquiry, as we had never discussed the case (and there is no record of any discussion in the minutes of the meetings of the division). In fact, when Jean telephoned me on 27 September, Gordon Bourne had already formally agreed to assess the case.

Monday, 26 September 1984. Dr Jean Richards to Gordon Bourne:

> Mr Cumberlege [the Chairman of Tower Hamlets Health Authority] has asked me to say how grateful he is that you have agreed to assess the papers relating to this case and advise him whether there is a *prima facie* case for suspension. The case notes are in my office if you wish to peruse them.

From the correspondence introduced at the enquiry, it is clear that some verbal discussion had taken place between Mr Bourne and someone from Tower Hamlets Health Authority before 26 September, and looking at the evidence of Gordon Bourne at the enquiry, the possibility that this person was Professor Grudzinskas cannot be discounted.

It is interesting that suspension was mentioned at this early stage. HM (61)112 is the circular which sets out how the Health Authority should proceed if a doctor's competence is questioned. It requires the District or Regional Health Officer to collect evidence and present a case to the Chairman of the Health Authority. If, having taken all appropriate advice, he then decides there is a *prima facie* case of incompetence, he must then present the case to the doctor for his or her comments.

Suspension, on the other hand, is normally used only as an emergency procedure when a doctor suddenly becomes dangerous to patients, because of mental illness or addiction to drugs or alcohol. The mention of this step in Jean Richards' letter indicates that the possibility was in the minds of both herself and the chairman from an early stage.

The role of the regional assessor

There are fourteen regional assessors, appointed by the DHSS to examine the case histories of women who die during pregnancy, labour or the puerperium (the period immediately following child-birth).

Every three years, these men produce reports called Confidential Enquiries into Maternal Mortality, a successful attempt by obstetricians to look at their practice and improve services for women. The regional assessor's role in deciding whether there was a *prima facie* case for an enquiry under HM (61)112 would be pivotal. His report would be the sole basis for my suspension. It was, therefore, crucial to ensure that the person who performed the task of assessing my management of the five cases could not possibly be influenced (even unconsciously) by bias and that he was representative of 'mainstream' views in the obstetric field.

Gordon Bourne was a senior consultant at St Bartholomew's Hospital. Francis Cumberlege, in his affidavit sworn in August 1985, describes him as 'a man of very great experience and distinction in obstetrics, indeed he is of world reputation. By reason of his position as regional assessor, he appeared then, and appears to me now the proper choice to advise the Health Authority.'

Gordon Bourne has a large private practice in Harley Street, and is best known for his popular book on pregnancy. The *Observer* was to describe him later, in an article about the enquiry, as 'a well-known exponent of the father knows best school'; and a senior member of the RCOG has described him as 'an arch conservative' in obstetric practice.

Gordon Bourne was indeed well known, and perhaps particularly for his views on that aspect of maternity care which formed the crux of the allegations against me – the circumstances in which a Caesarean section should be performed. His conservative approach put him at one end of the medical spectrum on the delivery of breech births – he believed they should be dealt with surgically.

I pointed out to Jean the reasons why Gordon Bourne was not the most suitable person to give an independent assessment. It is strange that the health authority should have viewed Gordon

Bourne as an impartial assessor. We shared a joint obstetric department with his at Bart's, and he knew both the professor, whom he had helped to train and whose approach to obstetrics he favoured more than mine, and myself. One could argue that although his job was to arbitrate between us, it would be difficult for him to be impartial.

Thursday, 4 October 1984
After Jean Richards had mentioned to me in passing that she was looking for the case notes of Baby U and was thinking of sending them to Gordon Bourne, I made an appointment to see her. She cancelled, on the grounds that the papers (on Mrs U) were not ready. Feeling very anxious, I went to see Mike Floyer and expressed my disquiet. He was friendly and reassuring, and said that he would be able to tell me more the following week.

But that same day Mike formally met Francis Cumberlege, Jean Richards, Sotiris Argyrou and Terry Dibiey (Regional Legal Adviser) to discuss whether the U case provided *prima facie* evidence for proceeding to an HM (61)112 enquiry. The decision to send Professor Grudzinskas' reports to Gordon Bourne was taken at that meeting.

Friday, 12 October 1984
The dean reassured me again, saying that 'one case was not enough for a 112', but later in the conversation he mentioned in passing that there were 'others in the pipeline'. By this time I had asked a senior manager in the health service – a former Tower Hamlets district administrator – about the HM (61)112 procedure. He said that even if a doctor was not competent, it was almost impossible to 'get' him; and since I clearly *was* competent, I had nothing to worry about.

During the summer, the professor had asked me for case reports on two more women. Professor Grudzinskas told me he needed the first report, on a woman named Linda Ganderson, to defend me against 'gossip' amongst my colleagues. The second case, that of Denise Lewis, was apparently needed because of criticisms of my administrative arrangements for study leave. The professor said my registrar had not known where I was or what to do, and that David Oram had not known he was standing in for me. I provided the professor with a case report detailing the comprehensive verbal and written arrangements which I had made for the study leave. In conversation I told him of the daily telephone calls with my staff during the period I was away and the case notes showed that I was in constant touch with the staff. Both these cases were, I thought, satisfactorily dealt with before August.

As well as this succession of demands for case reports (which were not within the professor's remit as my academic, but not clinical, superior) I had weekly letters from him about teaching, research, staff, the contingency fund, and the abortion service. Whatever the intention behind them, I saw these together as continuing the pressure on me which had begun with the letters threatening my dismissal.

I knew that I was not incompetent, and that my differences with my colleagues stemmed from a difference in approach and attitude. Although I was determined to continue providing what I believed were the right sort of obstetric services for women, I felt that in time, once the centralisation of obstetrics took place, we would all learn to work together. Hempsons, who had seen the three case reports I had produced for the professor, told me that these things were always happening and they blew over.

Looking back, now that I have all the letters assembled, and the time to study them in depth, it seems almost unbelievable that I could not have understood what was going on. I think this is partly because, having worked in five countries with three different professors, I had never come across a situation like this before. I was also very busy and I tended to write my letters to the MDU or Hempsons late at night when I had finished what I considered to be my real work – looking after patients and teaching students.

Monday, 15 October 1984. Dr Jean Richards to Gordon Bourne:

1. Mr Dibley [legal adviser] felt that you ought to be warned that the opinion which we have asked you to produce for the Chairman may be shown to Mrs Savage if the Chairman, as a result of that opinion, decides that there is a *prima facie* case for which an enquiry should proceed.
2. Professor Grudzinskas is investigating 3 further cases about which there is some concern. It is felt that you may wish to wait until you receive details of those before you produce your final letter for the Chairman.

I have been advised by Mr Dibley that Mrs Savage does not need to see any of the documentation so far until the Chairman makes the decision as to the existence or not of the *prima facie* case. I am, therefore, seeing her, but not showing her any of the letters which you have already received.

Thank you so much for your help.

Jean Richards never did see me, having cancelled the appointment I made in early October. The first time I saw this letter was when it was exhibited at the enquiry.

Tuesday, 30 October 1984. Professor Gedis Grudzinskas to Dr Jean Richards:

. . . I enclose my comments on three cases, in addition to another, which has been brought to my attention, for your information.

Regretfully, I am currently conducting an investigation into another case.

This case was Carol Lefevre, another woman whom I had allowed a trial of labour. Presumably he accepted my clinical judgement in this case as no report went on to Mr Bourne about her. Her healthy twins have appeared on many demonstrations and in newspapers since my suspension. She was delighted to have been allowed to have a trial of labour, even though she had a Caesarean section in the end.

Wednesday, 21 November 1984

I wrote to Hempsons, having learnt that the professor had acquired the notes of some of my patients, none of whom had complained about my care, before I'd even had the chance to do the reports he'd requested. I was advised to cooperate with the professor's requests and to deal with him by 'telephone rather than letter'.

Wednesday, 14 December 1984

Another request from the professor for me to provide detailed reports, this time of my handling of gynaecological cases. Producing these reports was extraordinarily time-consuming, and then and in subsequent months I expressed my exasperation to Mike Floyer at this waste of my time. I was astonished when a casual conversation with him revealed that, having spoken with Professor Grudzinskas, he had the (false) impression that the uterus of one of my patients had been perforated during an operation. I reported this to Hempsons, saying that I thought this was damaging to me.

My main concerns during this period were the continuing disagreements about the future of services for women within the department of obstetrics, my clinical work, which had continued to increase as GPs referred more women to me (between 1981 and 1984 the number of pregnant women in my care rose from 500 to 740 per annum), and my teaching and research commitments.

The reorganisation of the health service in 1982 and the cuts had added to the usual pressures, having a particularly severe effect on secretarial services. Poorly paid full-time posts were increasingly filled by temporary staff from agencies. During 1984 I had seven temporary secretaries. This meant I could never be sure that notes would be chased, results followed up and summaries prepared, unless I checked these details personally. It wasn't until I was suspended that I had time to realise that I had been routinely working eighty hours a week in order to deal properly with my clinical and academic work, committees outside the London Hospital, and the increasingly burdensome correspondence with the MDU.

My fellow consultants continued to work with me. There was no attempt to prevent me carrying on with teaching, treating patients and operating. No formal warning had been issued to this 'dangerous' clinician in the six months since baby U died. I was still unaware of the nature or extent of Gordon Bourne's investigation. (By now, he was examining five cases.) It would be another five months before I was suspended, and until then I remained in ignorance of the case being prepared against me.

In the first three months of 1985 both the District Medical Officer and the Chairman of the Health Authority urged Mr Bourne to produce his report on my management.

Tuesday, 15 January 1985. Francis Cumberlege to Gordon Bourne:

You will, of course, know the routine that the first task is for me, as Chairman, to establish that there is a *prima facie* case. Your report on the cases referred to would help me in reaching my conclusion . . . I wondered when I could expect your report.

As an experienced chairman one would have expected him to say 'to establish *whether* or not there is a *prima facie* case', particularly as he must have realised the importance of taking a scrupulously impartial and objective approach.

Wednesday, 27 March 1985. Dr Jean Richards to Gordon Bourne:

> [are you] yet in a position to submit your report . . . the chairman is most anxious for progress to be made in this matter as soon as possible.

In fact, in February 1985, Gordon Bourne had produced a draft report on the five cases. He later told the enquiry that he had meant to send the draft report to the Medical Defence Union, but his secretary had sent it to Dr Richards by mistake. What happened to the draft report in the next few weeks is a mystery. Gordon Bourne told the enquiry panel that he did not have all the correspondence as his filing cabinet had been cleared out when he retired from Bart's. From her letter to Gordon Bourne of 27 March, Dr Richards appeared to be unaware of the existence of the report.

Wednesday, 3 April 1985. Francis Cumberlege to Gordon Bourne:

> Months go by without a decision about Mrs Savage and I feel that further delay is damaging. I wondered if you are now in a position to let me have your report. ˙

Damaging to whom? The patients were not complaining.

Perhaps he meant that the credibility of the case for suspension would be damaged if a whole year had elapsed between the 'dangerous' event and any action being taken.

Gordon Bourne Sends his Final Reports to Dr J. Richards

At the enquiry, it was possible to compare Gordon Bourne's draft reports on 11 February with the final versions which were produced in April. Although most of the material and the main recommendations are identical, it appears from internal evidence that the February reports were compiled largely on the basis of summaries of each case prepared by Professor Grudzinskas rather than from the case notes themselves. At the enquiry Mr Bourne was to state that he had partial photocopies of the case notes when he wrote the first draft of his reports, but had not seen the original notes. My secretary was asked to provide three of the relevant case records, apparently for Professor Grudzinskas, on 28 February, while I was on leave. Before finalising his reports, Mr Bourne saw the original of the mothers' notes in at least four cases. His final report, dated 9 April, produced after nearly six months, consisted of eleven short pages, distilled from some 550 pages of medical notes.

On the basis of this document Francis Cumberlege decided to suspend me, bringing to an abrupt halt the work to which I had devoted my entire adult life.

> *Friday, 19 April 1985. Dr Richards to Gordon Bourne:*
>
> The Chairman joins me in offering you our sincere thanks for the enormous amount of work you have put into the reports recently submitted.
>
> The Chairman has decided that these provide a *prima facie* case for suspension under Section 112 of the 1961 Act, and Mrs Savage is being suspended from her Honorary Clinical Contract. The College will then decide whether to suspend her from College activities for which she is totally paid by them. Following submission of the evidence to her, and her replies, the necessity for a full enquiry will be decided upon.
>
> I would be grateful if you could submit a fee which would be appropriate for us to reimburse your time and expenses.
>
> Please may I thank you again for all the work you have put into this problem.

Mr Bourne waived his fee.

· CHAPTER 5 ·

The Muted Response of the Medical Establishment

I will maintain the honour and noble tradition of the medical profession. A clinician shall behave towards his colleagues as he would have them behave towards him. A clinician shall deal honestly with patients and colleagues and strive to expose those physicians who engage in fraud and deception.

Geneva code of ethics for the medical profession

I was not simply a doctor: I also taught medical students at the London Hospital Medical College, part of London University. When I was suspended I assumed my academic colleagues would support me. On the day following the suspension of my honorary clinical contract, I received the following letter

25 April 1985. Professor Grudzinskas to Wendy Savage:

Dear Wendy,
I regret that following a discussion with Dr Jean Richards this morning concerning suspension of your Honorary Consultant Contract, I think it is in your interest and the interest of the Medical College that you should be withdrawn from all teaching and research activities in Obstetrics and Gynaecology in relation to under- and postgraduate student teaching until resolution of the present situation.
    I wish this to take effect forthwith.
Yours sincerely,
JG Grudzinskas

Mr Leigh dictated a letter in reply that I took in to the college that night. He advised against writing to the Academic Board but sent a copy to the dean.

26 April 1985. Hempsons to Professor Grudzinskas:

We have been instructed by the Medical Defence Union and their member, Mrs W. D. Savage, with regard to your letter of the 25th April. In that letter you assert your view that it is in our client's interest that she should be 'withdrawn' from teaching and research activities in relation to under- and postgraduate student teaching until resolution of the present situation. Our client does not agree.

You also said that it is your opinion that it is in the interest of the Medical College that this should be so. You do not say why this may be. You will be aware that for a doctor of our client's standing to be suspended from an academic post without notice and for no more precise reason than that it is 'in the interest of the Medical College' is gravely damaging. All our client's rights with regard to this step are reserved. In the hope that the damage which follows from this can be limited, we request you to withdraw the suspension forthwith.

In the event that you decline to withdraw our client's suspension we should be grateful if you would explain precisely why it is in the interest of the Medical College so that we can advise our client further as to the remedies available to her . . .

We are sending a copy of this letter to the dean.

Yours sincerely,

Hempsons

As Mr Leigh finished dictating this he told me that this letter virtually told the professor that he might be sued for libel and I felt cheered that at least I would be able to teach whilst I endured the suspension from my clinical work.

The Threat to Academic Freedom

At the Academic Board meeting on 29 April the 'suspension from clinical duties' of an un-named senior lecturer was announced 'sadly' by Professor Blandy as an addition to the routine report of the Academic Division of Surgery, of which I was a member. Professor Grudzinskas then said he 'deeply regretted this matter' and the dean clinched the identification when he said that the college would continue to pay *her* salary.

The dean added that the matter was *sub judice* and could not therefore be discussed. (Francis Cumberlege later prevented discussion at a DHA meeting by asserting that my case was *sub judice*. This effectively closed off other avenues of approach and ensured a major public confrontation. In fact, *sub judice* was used incorrectly in the context of my suspension, and there was no legal reason why my case could not be discussed openly.)

That night several people phoned wanting to know what on earth I could have done that was so dreadful as to require my suspension. Seducing the patients? Embezzling NHS funds? I replied that I had been suspended for alleged incompetence, but that no, I hadn't killed dozens of patients. Following Hempsons' advice, I said nothing more. It was a strange feeling being under suspicion like this and I felt sad that people would doubt my competence after all those years of working in the same hospital. Some of them had recommended me to their wives. Did they regret that now? Did they think they had had a lucky escape?

In the hospital the next day I noticed how some people did not look at me as we passed in the corridor. Some even crossed the street rather than have to speak to me. Part of me felt hurt; another part saw that it was very useful to see who was and who was not going to support me in the coming battle.

At the Academic Division of Surgery meeting on 1 May I read out a statement in which I denied the allegations of incompetence and said I would fight to restore my good name and professional reputation. I insisted that this be minuted and included in the report to the Academic Board and this was agreed by the chairman.

Many people expressed concern about the way I had been banned from teaching. It established a precedent, as although professors have overall responsibility for the direction of teaching, in practice the individual academic is free to present the subject matter as she or he sees fit and the concept of freedom of thought and speech is jealously guarded in universities in Great Britain. They were also disturbed by the fact that this had been announced to the Academic Board without consultation with the division or myself. Professor Blandy defended himself by saying it was the dean's decision but, 'if one of my chaps was operating badly it would be ludicrous to let him teach Academic Urology'. He gathered his papers and left.

It seemed I was to be assumed guilty until proven innocent. I continued to go into work and eat in the Medical College Blizard Club lunch room; I was not going to allow people to think that I was ashamed of my actions, or act as if I was guilty of these charges.

I received more than twenty letters of support from GPs and midwives in the first four days after my suspension. Yet after the Academic Board meeting, only a handful of hospital doctors and Medical College staff wrote to me. The contrast was striking.

The medical students were very upset by my suspension. Several of them joined the Support Group and helped with the march even though finals were approaching. They had a noticeboard in the common room where they put press cuttings about my campaign. Later they asked me to give them some lectures before finals. They found a school hall near the college and I was encouraged by the large number who attended. The dean told them, after a routine lecture, that it was to 'save Mrs Savage from emotional trauma' that I had been asked not to teach. His words were greeted with incredulous laughter.

Between June 1985 and February 1986 I wrote six letters to the Academic Board, appealing to my professional colleagues to support my request to be allowed to continue to teach students. In October the Board voted not to support my request by seventeen votes to twelve.

The Royal College of Obstetricians and Gynaecologists

The irony of receiving the highest award to a member of my profession, the Fellowship of the Royal College of Obstetricians and Gynaecologists, came home to me when, suspended from my post, I attended the award ceremony in June.

Each year the fellows are circulated with papers inviting them to name people whom they consider deserving of fellowship status. Acceptance is not automatically granted but is awarded by a Fellowship Committee for 'advancing the science and practice of obstetrics and gynaecology'. Of the 764 consultant obstetricians and gynaecologists in England and Wales, there are eighty-eight women (11.5 per cent). This is reflected within the committee structure of the RCOG where 10 per cent of the members are women. However, in 1986 only one woman was elected to the council, and all but one of the twenty-six committees are chaired by men. Male members and fellows are invited to join two clubs, the Travellers and the Gynaecological Club, and membership is limited. Excluded from the cosy male get-togethers where, it is rumoured, all the consultant posts are 'fixed', women have formed their own club but it does not seem to be an effective pressure group for women, either as obstetricians or as patients. The incongruity of a specialty devoted to women being almost totally controlled by men has always struck me forcefully.

The official position of the RCOG is that it represents the

interest of all members and fellows and must remain neutral in disputes. Its position of not taking sides meant that the 'Savage' case has never been mentioned officially in its newsletters. On a personal level, senior council officers have been supportive towards me, and I was told informally at the highest level that they would have been happy to sit down with the obstetricians at Tower Hamlets to try to find some way forward. Nevertheless the college declined to comment on what it termed 'the difficulties' until a conclusion had been reached.

The General Medical Council

Through the General Medical Council, which has almost one hundred members, both appointed and elected, the medical profession sets its own standards and disciplines its own members.

One of the most important principles of the practice of medicine is that of clinical autonomy, which allows a fully trained doctor the responsibility for deciding which mode of treatment is best for his or her patients. In practice, clinical autonomy means that consultants and GPs are of equal status, are responsible for their own clinical decisions and should not be criticised by their colleagues as long as these decisions are 'within the broad limits of acceptable medical practice'. The GMC's handbook also states that the deprecation by a doctor of the professional skill, knowledge, qualifications or services of another doctor could amount to serious professional misconduct.

Throughout the time that Professor Grudzinskas was asking me for case reports I had maintained to the MDU and Hempsons that he had no right to ask me for these reports as he was not my clinical superior.

I decided to raise the matter with the president of the GMC.

17 November 1985. Wendy Savage to Sir John Walton:

At the moment I am not seeking to lay a complaint against my colleagues at the London Hospital, but am seeking your advice about matters of interprofessional relationships which do not seem to be covered by the 'Blue Book', but which I had thought were part of the code of practice between doctors.

Firstly, I believe that doctors holding either honorary or normal NHS consultant contracts are independent consultants in their own right and that, whilst a professor is academically superior to a senior lecturer, as far as clinical matters are concerned, he has no more right to criticise or direct a senior lecturer than one of his NHS colleagues.

Secondly, is it ethical to ask for case reports from a colleague in order 'to defend you against gossip' and then use these cases to boost a complaint via the HM 61/112 procedure?

Thirdly, is it usual for another consultant to order notes belonging to one of his colleagues in order to prepare case reports about clinical care, without the knowledge and consent of that person and in the absence of a complaint by a patient or formal enquiry of which the department is aware?

Fourthly, I enclose a letter which, as you can see, was widely circulated within the hospital, was not marked private and confidential, and which I was advised was not libellous, despite the fact that parts of it are untrue, because it was 'privileged'. Does the GMC concern itself with matters of this nature?

Weeks passed and there was no reply, so on 21 December I wrote again, having by now seen the statements made by my colleagues in preparation for the forthcoming enquiry. On 6 January 1986, I received a reply and an apology for the delay from Sir John Walton. In essence, he confirmed that academics did have clinical autonomy, and referring to the pamphlet 'Professional Conduct and Discipline: Fitness to Practise' that doctors would normally only disclose confidential information about patients to other doctors who are looking after or taking over responsibility for that patient, he continued:

I would not normally think it proper for a doctor to take an initiative in disclosing confidential information about one of his or her patients to another doctor for any other purpose, unless that was a purpose covered by other aspects of the Council's guidance, such as disclosure at the order of a judge or other presiding officers of a court. Similarly, I would not regard it as usual practice for a doctor to request access to the clinical notes of another doctor's patient for any other purpose other than one of those mentioned in the Council's guidance; any doctor who does so and who discloses the information so obtained should therefore be prepared to justify his action, in accordance with paragraph (3) of the Council's guidance.

The Official Hospital Response

In February 1985 Sam Cohen, Professor of Psychiatry, became

Chairman of the Final Medical Committee and Medical Council. He is a quietly spoken man who has always been pleasant to me. I made an appointment to see him the week after I was suspended and told him briefly about the five cases. I said that even if I were incompetent it seemed to me that my suspension raised questions that needed to be discussed, not just for me, but for all doctors at the London. These were the use of suspension before I had been given a chance to defend myself and the secretive way the case had been built up. Sam was shocked by my suspension and expressed his support for me.

I wrote to Professor Cohen after the DHA on 9 May 1985 had not agreed to my request for the suspension to be lifted and Mr Cumberlege had said publicly that an enquiry was going ahead:

> I enclose the letter [see Ch. 4, p. 41] which started off the enquiry process under the HM (61)112 procedure, which could lead to my dismissal. Unless I accept the charges of mismanagement, which I do not, the next stage, after I have replied formally to the DMO within twenty-eight days from 24.4.85, is a formal enquiry with two obstetricians and a legally qualified chairman.

I then went into details of the U case, the 'worst' of the five which I allegedly mismanaged. I ended the letter:

> It was then alleged, in retrospect, that my registrar who had delivered the baby, had done so badly, and that a tentorial tear had resulted. This is an extremely rare occurrence in a term baby delivered by Caesarean section. What I am being condemned for is allowing the woman to have a trial of labour with a scar in the uterus and a breech presentation. Both the woman and her husband wanted her to try and deliver vaginally, and declined the offer of a Caesarean section twice during the labour.
>
> *At neither time did I consider that the baby's condition was such that I should force the couple to agree to an operation* and this is a matter of clinical judgement. There was no post-mortem at the couple's request.
>
> I do not think that this is the way one expects one's colleagues to behave and I also think that the Chairman of the Health Authority has been poorly advised.
>
> The result will be bad publicity for the hospital and the college which I regret.

I had copied this letter to two people whom I knew would speak in my defence at the FMC meeting on 16 May 1985. (The FMC is made up of the chairmen of the hospital divisions and meets monthly. In addition all consultants are members of the Medical Council which meets three times a year. The same person chairs both bodies.) There was considerable discussion and concern about how I could have been suspended without the chair of the FMC knowing about it, and the damage being done to the hospital by the publicity which had already occurred. The committee asked Professor Cohen to speak to Mr Cumberlege.

What passed between them I do not know, but Mr Cumberlege was not swayed by the opinions of the hospital consultants expressed through the chair of the FMC.

Between June and August I asked members of the Medical Council to raise the manner in which I had been suspended. I was disappointed not to be invited to the June meeting; nor did they discuss the matter because the debate 'might have got out of hand' and 'people might say things they regret later'. Most people apparently thought that nothing could be discussed until I was reinstated. At the July meeting of the FMC the committee asked its chair to see again if there was any way of resolving the matter; Professor Cohen wrote to me, the Chairman of the Division of Obstetrics and Gynaecology and the Chairman of the Health Authority to offer the services of senior medical staff. I replied as follows on 31 July 1985:

Dear Sam,

Thank you for your letter and offer to help in any way possible.

I certainly would welcome anything that could be done to make it possible for us to work effectively and harmoniously in the Department of Obstetrics and Gynaecology.

At present affidavits have been prepared and my solicitor tells me that the case should be lodged with the High Court on Monday, 5.8.85.

Two professors and one reader have said that the five cases were not sufficient material to suspend me and two of them said that any enquiry into the two they thought did show errors of management should include the whole department. We are suing for reinstatement on the grounds that my suspension was unlawful and a breach of my contract.

Any steps that could be taken to make reinstatement as painless as possible for everybody concerned I would welcome. The latest offer from Professor Grudzinskas through an intermediary is 'if WDS will resign we will drop all the charges', so I find it difficult to see a way forward in the present climate and with court proceedings almost inevitable.

I deeply regret the divisions in our department that taking evidence from the junior staff will almost certainly bring. I wonder if your good offices could be used to assist them to make the difficult decisions that will be forced on them? I understand that the DMO has now written to say that as the notes could not be released they should be perused in her office and the doctors' report on their personal involvement be prepared there. I have advised the junior staff to discuss this with their defence societies, but perhaps they would like to talk to someone from outside of the department as well . . .

Thank you again for your offer of help.

In August no FMC meeting is held and by September it was known that the High Court case for immediate reinstatement had been lost and that an enquiry would take place in November.

In October, I was refused permission to attend the Medical Council meeting the next day. That night was one of the 'low spots' in the time since my suspension. It seemed that the – as I saw it – male professional view was that having been unjustly accused I had to accept this injustice and await the slow creaking HM (61)112 enquiry procedure, however much it cost the NHS or me personally. If I gave up and threw in the sponge it would show that I wasn't tough enough to stand the pace of a teaching hospital consultant life. In a way I felt that many people hoped that I would give up and then the whole affair could be smoothed over and forgotten and people would not have to face the fact that those they worked with, referred patients to, or drank tea with in the consultants' room, had behaved in such an unusual way.

At that point I thought that I would stop trying to get my hospital colleagues to act.

· CHAPTER 6 ·

The Public Protests

Off stage there have been unedifying antics. Some doctors who complain about 'trial by the media' seem to find nothing repugnant in 'trial by gossip'.

Michael O'Donnell, *British Medical Journal*, 14 September 1985

In the months following my suspension the position of the medical establishment became clear to me. Meanwhile, however, my case had aroused enormous national interest and concern.

Word of my suspension had travelled quickly. The news certainly reached some organisations before I was formally suspended. It seems that a health visitor, pregnant and booked under my care, had overheard a conversation between a midwife and a GP after a lunchtime meeting. She was so shocked that she immediately rang Sue Hadley, the Tower Hamlets National Childbirth Trust (NCT) teacher, whom I knew slightly. They agreed that this outrageous action should be fought and even before my meeting with Jean Richards they had rung the NCT national office. The NCT then informed the press.

At the time, I was still in a state of shock. I had not thought about publicity. I still hoped that the MDU and Hempsons would somehow get an injunction to stop what was so obviously unjust and wrong. In retrospect, although I would have preferred to inform the press on my own terms, it was probably just as well that it was done for me. In less than twenty-four hours, doctors, midwives, a neighbouring Health Authority member, the Community Health Council and medical correspondents from the national newspapers had all left messages on my answerphone.

The Local GPs Respond

On Thursday, the professor told the GP representatives on the Maternity Services Liaison Committee (MSLC) that I had been suspended. Unknown to me, on Friday evening, forty-eight hours after my suspension, local GPs and midwives gathered at South Poplar Health Centre, one of the four practices I visited as part of the community obstetric scheme. Fifteen GPs came, including several of the older ones, like Dr Bernard Taylor who had been in practice for thirty-five years in the East End and Dr Nebhrajani, speaking on behalf of Asian women. They decided to form a committee, later to become the Appeal Fund. Mary Edmondson, Tony Jewell and David Widgery were elected as members.

Mary Edmondson had had both of her two young children at Mile End. I had worked with Tony Jewell at the Mile End when he was Peter Huntingford's Senior House Officer and I had looked after his wife during both her pregnancies. She was then due to have her second baby in three weeks' time. Several of the younger GPs had done their vocational training at the London, as had Tony Jewell, and had either worked for Peter Huntingford or myself.

I am told that it was their contact with me at a clinical level as GPs, and their respect for the support I had tried to give them as professionals (both in providing the kind of care that they wanted for their patients, and in encouraging them to take on more antenatal and intrapartum maternity care) which made them act. Many had small children and as young GPs were still building up their practices. Writing and circulating petitions, and later writing and talking to the newspaper, TV and radio journalists was a heavy and time-consuming burden for them all, and I am grateful to them for that invaluable support.

The many doctors who say to me, 'But how could you go back and work in Tower Hamlets after your colleagues have attacked you like this?' perhaps do not realise that sixty-eight of the eighty-three GPs in Tower Hamlets signed that first rushed petition which the GP Committee presented to the Chairman of the District Health Authority. They continued to support me throughout this long struggle – even though, initially, they knew nothing about the details of the cases. They knew, however, that I was not incompetent. In many ways GPs are in a better position to judge competence, as they are responsible for the long-term care of patients and have more contact with consultants than consultants often have with each other.

On 6 May, Bank Holiday Monday, the GP Committee, now with the addition of Dr Jo Shawcross from the third practice I visited, met and planned a small press conference to be held on the 9th (the day of the monthly District Health Authority's next meeting) at Steele's Lane Health Centre.

The DHA meeting was ·packed. Around sixty people turned up, in small groups or on their own initiative, to demand my reinstatement. Beverley Beech of AIMS (the Association for Improvements in the Maternity Services) collected their names.

Mary Edmondson presented the GPs' letter calling for my reinstatement and also presented a petition from the medical students describing me as 'an inspired and conscientious teacher' – despite the 7.45 a.m. ward rounds! A further petition from the Mile End Hospital had been signed by 150 people from all grades of staff.

The Wendy Savage Support Group

The Wendy Savage Support Group was formally launched on 16 May 1985, in the basement of a local community centre in Bethnal Green. More than fifty people were crammed into the room – GPs, midwives, nurses, medical students, local mothers, and a few fathers, and representatives of the national consumer movements like AIMS which, through Beverley Beech, had been active from the day of my suspension. Sue Hadley and Heather Reid attended for the NCT and Christine Smith and Ron Brewer represented the Community Health Council, the NHS watchdog group for patients. There were women from the Maternity Services Liaison Committee which is a link group between women from ethnic minorities and the antenatal service. Many of the women were former patients of mine. They decided to hold a march on 13 June, the day of the next Health Authority meeting, and to write individually and collectively to Mr Cumberlege and other people in positions of authority.

Posters were printed and badges produced with the slogan 'Wendy's Best – Investigate the Rest' and 'The Savage Cut – Who Asked Us?' Car stickers showing a baby with the slogan 'Reinstate Wendy Savage Now' were provided free of charge by Malcolm Crowe, whose wife had chosen to have her first baby at home with my blessing, and had been looked after by Mary Edmondson.

The public response was overwhelming. Women stood in street

markets, toddlers at their feet, collecting signatures for petitions. Petitions went around nursery schools, GPs' surgeries and Labour Party meetings. Vast numbers of posters advertising the march appeared all over the borough virtually overnight – on hoardings, bus-stops, in clinics and libraries, and in the windows of people's homes.

Both Beverley Beech and Sheila Kitzinger of the NCT were veteran campaigners for women's rights in childbirth, and using their connections the Support Group added to the national media coverage of the issue. Sheila's article, 'Battle of the Birth Rights', in the *Sunday Times* on 19 May and pieces in *New Society* and the *New Statesman* carried news of the march. The *East London Advertiser*, the *Guardian, Hospital Doctor* (distributed free to all doctors working in NHS hospitals) and the *Nursing Times* all carried features about different aspects of the case and the campaign for my reinstatement.

Taking the advice of Hempsons, I was refusing to speak to the press, concentrating my efforts on the hospital and Medical College in the hope of an internal solution. I spent my time conferring with Mr Leigh, my solicitor, drafting letters, gathering statistics and dictating notes on the five cases.

At the time, I was not aware of the immense efforts of my supporters behind the scenes and it was only later that I realised, with gratitude, their work on my behalf.

As the press coverage widened, letters of support flooded in daily and I began to question the lawyers' advice to avoid publicity. On 28 May, five weeks after my suspension, I decided to change my solicitors. Although I had no reason to doubt their integrity, I had been feeling, increasingly, that Hempsons were part of the same medical establishment which I felt was attacking me. Mr Leigh was on first name terms with Mr Dibley, the Health Authority's solicitor, and I realised that they were usually on the same side, defending doctors against patients. I, on the other hand, was supported by my patients against some of my fellow doctors.

Helena Kennedy, a barrister, had recommended Brian Raymond, of Bindman and Partners, to me. He had just success-fully defended Clive Ponting in the 'Belgrano Secrets' trial. He had time to take the case, and I went to meet him the next day.

I drove to Bindman's offices in Finsbury Park. The contrast could not have been more marked. Bindman and Partners are known for their interest in civil liberties and their staff reflected their principles. I went up a narrow staircase to the top floor; the office was small and functional, crammed with papers. Brian Raymond, shorter and less angular than Mr Leigh, was in his shirtsleeves in the sunny, uncurtained room. The atmosphere was relaxed and informal. I immediately felt at ease and although it was painful having to go through the details of the suspension and its aftermath again, I knew I had made the right decision. Brian's view was that rather than shunning the publicity, I should use it to my best advantage.

I was still hesitant about using publicity, and although I had known since February that I was to be elected to the Fellowship of the Royal College of Obstetricians and Gynaecologists, I had kept quiet about it. It was therefore a surprise to me when I opened my *Guardian* on 1 June to read, 'Top Award for Suspended Doctor'. The article went on to describe how Professor Chamberlain, the junior vice-president of the RCOG, had publicly supported me. The solicitors, Hempsons, had asked him for a report on the five cases to be submitted to the District Health Authority. I knew he had seen the criticisms and the case notes, and felt doubly cheered by his stand.

On Sunday 2 June, Katherine Whitehorn's regular *Observer* column was headlined, 'Who's Hysterical Now?', referring to the medical establishment. Apparently an attempt to oust me, using 'mental instability' as an excuse, had been considered but rejected.

On Wednesday 5 June, I went to the Royal College to receive the award. I evaded the press photographers outside, leaving the taxi by another door. All the old photos in the press files were from the days when my hair had been long and straight so they didn't recognise me with my comparatively new hairstyle. Instead they beseiged my stepmother, under the mistaken impression that she was me.

On 7 June Brian Raymond and I had met with the Support Group for the first time. Although I wanted to go on the march we thought it best that I did not because its focus was the feeling of the *community* about the effect of my suspension on the women of Tower Hamlets. If I were there, the press and the District Health Authority could dismiss it as simply being a personal protest and this it was not. Three of my four children went. I dropped them outside the Mile End Hospital at 1.30 p.m. There was a handful of people there and I felt that anxiety I always feel when giving a party, when everything is prepared and the time for starting approaches, and I think no one will come. But more than a thousand people turned up, pushing prams and pushchairs. MPs Jo Richardson and Ian Mikardo, who had sponsored an Early Day motion in Parliament calling for my reinstatement, marched along with the Maternity Service Liaison workers, women from Bangladesh and Somalia and women's health organisations. Led by a small band, they marched from Mile End Hospital, along Whitechapel Road to the London Hospital, Whitechapel, where the DHA meeting was to be held. There the Assistant District Administrator was sent out to face the well-behaved crowd and its police escort, whilst Mr Cumberlege and Sotiris Argyrou kept a low profile. The Support Group had done a magnificent job. In four weeks they had organised a very big event, on a shoestring, and with no previous experience of doing anything quite like this. I learned afterwards that a senior professor, who had watched the march arriving from an upstairs window, remarked, 'Who would have thought to see the day a rabble marched on the London Hospital?' That's no rabble, I thought; those are your patients.

The next day's press coverage lifted my hopes even further. Several papers carried pieces about the march and over the weekend the *Observer* carried a feature on my suspension, following up a series of *New Statesman* articles which had investigated the medical-political background to the events and the extent of my colleagues' involvement in private practice. Francis Cumberlege's response to the protest was quoted by the *Observer* as, 'I was in the tea business: I was out in Bengal from 1946–1953. I don't want lectures from women on what Bengalis want.'

Because I had decided to leave Hempsons, it was estimated that I could face legal costs of around £50,000. Brian Raymond told me not to worry. When he had defended Clive Ponting people spontaneously sent money in without any public appeal from him.

Sam Smith, a seventy-six-year-old ex-Tower Hamlets GP, staunch socialist and a fighter for justice throughout his life, rang me on 8 June to say that he had been sent a cheque for £100 and suggested that an appeal fund should be set up. He embarked on an enthusiastic one-man telephone campaign to local GPs, which raised several hundred pounds. Then a group of GPs took on the extra work involved by forming the Appeal Fund Committee. The press coverage of the High Court hearings in August and September mentioned that I had to pay my own legal fees. The public response was astounding. By mid-September the fund had reached £2,000; by mid-October £5,000, and by the time the official circular asking for donations was printed, it stood at £9,000. Eventually the Appeal Fund was to reach £60,000.

The gulf between what women were seeking in obstetric care and what the medical profession wanted to provide became clear from the different responses of the community and the medical establishment. The doctors and health workers who worked in the Tower Hamlets Health District were willing to become publicly involved in my case because they knew, and liked, the kind of care I provided – and that I was competent. Their public declaration of support gave me strength. They and the women's health organisations who were involved from the beginning of my suspension ensured that my case caught the attention of the media: my case was no longer the fight of the individual for her livelihood but a focus for a countrywide debate on the future delivery of maternity services.

The strength of feeling about the case and the whole issue of maternity services must have surprised my colleagues and taken the medical establishment by surprise. Many doctors were horrified at the prospect of the profession washing its dirty linen in public. From the beginning, when the chairman of the Health Authority declared the matter *sub judice* and the professional bodies refused to become involved, it was clear that their overriding concern in my case was for a discreet and private conclusion to the affair. The public silence of my consultant colleagues contrasted strongly with the willingness of many of them to talk behind the scenes. One journalist said to me after some days of talking to doctors: 'I've come to the conclusion that if I said to a doctor, "Do you put on a gown and gloves to operate?" he would say, "Off-record, yes."'

Gossip thrived in the corridors not only of the London Hospital but also amongst examiners for the Royal College of Obstetricians and Gynaecologists and members of the General Medical Council. Michael O'Donnell, the well-known medical journalist, writing in the *British Medical Journal* in May 1986, said:

Some doctors who complain vociferously about trial by the media
are themselves active proponents of that traditional medical
pastime, trial by gossip. During the Savage case I decided to
document this practice by noting items of gossip that were offered to
me or passed on in my presence, and then investigating them as best
I could to see if there was any substance to them.

I found it a depressing assignment. The gossip, for instance,
included allegations about Mrs Savage's sexual inclinations and
marital history which if those who uttered them had bothered to
make but the simplest of inquiries they would have learnt to be
untrue. Yet these personal smears were passed on in conversation
by some of the most senior people in medicine and accepted
unquestioned by others as evidence for the prosecution in the court
of gossip. There were also professional smears.

I intend to publish the full dossier one day but now offer one
example to advance my argument. Here is an excerpt from a letter I
wrote last November to a professor of obstetrics and gynaecology, a
man that I had enjoyed meeting and whose work I much admire:
'You may remember that, in conversation, I was interested in your
views on the "Wendy Savage case", and you said that "we have to
do something about someone who has cut six ureters".

'The conversation was private so I would never attribute the
remark to you but I've recently been examining the extent to which
our profession indulges in "trial by gossip" and have been trying to
find out just how true are some "received truths".

'It's taken a long time to track down the details – for reasons you
can easily guess – and, though I can't be certain, it seems likely that,
during Wendy Savage's time at the London, only two of her patients
have had "ureteric complications". One, operated on by her
registrar, had a ligature put round one branch of a congenital
double ureter; the other suffered ureteritis after a ligature had been
placed close to it but not around it.

'I don't expect you to tell me who told you about the six ureters
though I hope that you will have a chance to pass back this bit of
"counter information" and would be interested to know what his or
her reaction is.'

He eventually replied: 'It was very good of you to write. I have
asked around since you were in touch and, although the rumour
seems to be widespread, as you suggest, there is no real substance. I
think we all have learnt a lesson from this but unfortunately,
whatever the outcome, medicine, the practice of obstetrics, and the
individuals concerned in the London debacle cannot benefit.' And
so say all of us.

In the month following my suspension there were more than
twenty articles about it in the national and medical press. They
struck a chord with women all over the country who wrote in their

hundreds to explain that their own experience of birth had made them want a different kind of care. Regular press reports – particularly in the *Guardian* – throughout the fifteen months I was suspended, ensured that the issues were kept alive. Television and radio coverage, once I had decided to 'go public', helped me to reach millions of people. I made two rules for the media – I would not discuss my colleagues or the cases. I was only prepared to talk about the issues involved as I saw them: the provision of obstetric care, who makes the decisions and disciplinary procedures for doctors. The public campaign was, I believe, essential if justice was also to be a factor in the resolution to my suspension. But there was another, more important, aspect of the publicity. Women throughout the country have realised that they have the right and the power to see that the health services they get are the ones they want.

· CHAPTER 7 ·
The Legal Battle

Your power in the court is directly proportional to your power
outside the court.

Brian Raymond's advice to Wendy Savage when they first met

At the DHA meeting on 9 May 1985, Mr Cumberlege had said
publicly that an enquiry would go ahead, although I had, in
accordance with the circular HM(61)112, four weeks to reply to
the written criticisms of the five cases that Jean Richards had
handed me on 24 April. It took three of those weeks before the case
notes were sent to Hempsons. Whilst we were waiting for them, Mr
Leigh had told me that if 'safety' were mentioned in connection
with a 112, an enquiry was virtually certain to take place. In view
of this I decided not to reveal my defence. Hempsons wrote on 22
May to this effect, but no reply had been received when I decided
to change my solicitor a week later.

Brian Raymond and I decided that our first task was to see if the
DHA could be persuaded to change its mind about holding an
enquiry in view of the community support for me and mounting
public pressure.

Then, on Monday 3 June, Jean Richards phoned me to see if an
HM(61)112 enquiry could be avoided. I replied in writing that
while I must take every possible step to preserve my reputation and
career, which had already suffered as a result of the action taken by
the chairman of the DHA, I was prepared to forgo a public enquiry
providing certain conditions were met. On the assumption that a
final decision had not yet been made by the chairman as to whether
a *prima facie* case existed, I would assist him in making this decision
by putting forward my own account of these cases to an independent senior obstetrician of standing, from another district. He
would then advise as to the existence of a *prima facie* case of
professional incompetence on my part in relation to the five cases
taken in the context of my overall practice as a consultant since
1977.

Jean's reply was surprisingly swift, and the ground had changed somewhat. There had been 'a little bit of a misunderstanding', she wrote:

> My proposal was that you should sit down with one or two outside assessors from the Royal College and then *meet with our obstetricians to see if a* modus vivendi *was possible* (my emphasis). On that front I understand from the Royal College that they now feel that a reconciliation is not possible . . . In addition we now have the formal letter from Hempsons instructing us to proceed to . . . a 112 enquiry . . . I must point out that the enquiry is in private, not in public as you state in your letter . . .

What Jean had in fact suggested to me on the phone was that if I were to sit down with someone from the RCOG, herself and the chairman, maybe we could go through the case notes together and avoid a 112. The other obstetricians had never been mentioned.

On 5 June 1985, while I was having lunch after receiving my FRCOG, a senior official of the Royal College had told me that the district had in fact approached him with this idea on Monday but had withdrawn the suggestion on the Wednesday morning.

Brian wrote to all members of the District Health Authority on 11 June, just before the DHA meeting on the thirteenth. It was a long, four-page letter, and made several points:

1. We appreciated the responsibility the DHA had to provide services, and heed the advice of their medical advisers. However, they would also wish to be fair to any individual doctor whose competence had been challenged.

2. The evidence that came from patients, GPs, the RCOG and the perinatal figures we enclosed did not suggest that my competence was in doubt but rather that there were differences in opinion about the way that obstetrics was practised.

3. It was well known that there were differences of opinion between the obstetricians in the district.

4. Although the DMO had given me twenty-eight days, until 23 May, to respond to the criticisms, the chairman had announced publicly on 9 May that an enquiry was to take place in any event, and the dean confirmed this in a conversation with me on the eleventh. I had therefore reserved my defence, but if it was not the case that an enquiry was already scheduled, we were prepared to take part in a review of the cases to establish whether or not there

was a *prima facie* case. We suggested someone of the standing of one of the vice-presidents of the RCOG acting in a private capacity.

Brian's letter concluded:

> It will not be necessary to emphasise that this issue has aroused strong feelings in many quarters over the past few weeks, not least in Mrs Savage, who feels herself the subject of wholly unfounded allegations. At this stage, however, our purpose is to find a satisfactory resolution to the present situation, rather than to criticise those responsible for bringing it about. It is unfortunate that the Authority has become involved in what is clearly a dispute between practitioners over clinical practice and judgement, but having done so, we respectfully suggest that the matter can be dealt with most sensibly in the manner proposed above. At the same time we feel that it is only fair to point out that in the absence of a satisfactory resolution, at an early stage, Mrs Savage will be forced to protect her rights in this matter by means of action in the High Court, although this step would be taken with the greatest reluctance.

I had been pleased to find, when I had worked out the perinatal mortality figures for the London Hospital, that my rate was numerically the lowest, although with such small numbers the differences were not statistically significant. (A perinatal death occurs when a baby is stillborn or dies in the first week of life. The perinatal mortality rate, or PMR, is the number of deaths per 1,000 total births.) We had included a table giving these figures with the letter. The morning of 13 June, Jean Richards rang Brian and thanked him for the approach but said my perinatal figures were meaningless, comparing 'apples and pears'. Her argument was that I didn't get referrals or difficult cases at Mile End. In fact, I had checked on as many variables as possible which affected perinatal mortality, and told her so. 'But, anyway Wendy,' she said, 'it's not that your practice is dangerous . . . it's just that it is different from the others.' For a minute, I was completely speechless.

It was at this point that I made the biggest mistake of the whole campaign. Earlier that week, when talking to Eva Alberman, Professor of Clinical Epidemiology, she had asked me if Professor Dennis from Southampton would be a suitable person to review the cases. I respected his work in the Wessex region on abortion services, and knew he was one of the Regional Assessors in

Maternal Mortality. Eva said he had been suggested by the RCOG.

When Jean Richards rang me she put forward his name, and still thinking that we were going to sit down with the lawyers and the chairman to work out the exact way to do this review, using my considered responses to the allegation, I said I had no objection in principle to him. I did not know that Jean Richards had already sent the note, *with Gordon Bourne's adverse comments*, but without my considered responses on which I was still working, to John Dennis the previous evening.

I was taken aback to find a message from Professor Dennis on my answerphone that Saturday. On Wednesday 19 June I travelled to Southampton with the first draft of my comments about the five cases. John Dennis hardly looked at these but we had a long conversation. He was very sympathetic, and said he didn't agree with Gordon Bourne about most of the cases but he thought that with Mrs U, I-had had a brainstorm. I tried to explain my policy of allowing a woman to experience labour even if I think the chance of success is small, but I could see that this was a foreign concept to him. I also told him a little bit about the problems in the department and gave him the perinatal figures by consultant, including the variables of social class, age, parity, gestation at delivery, birthweight and serious medical illness. On the way back in the train, I felt relieved and reassured.

The next two weeks were hectic as Brian and I went through the case notes and translated my comments into legal language. By this time Brian had moved back to the head office of Bindman's, opposite King's Cross. We sat in his room over an amusement arcade. It was hot, and the tinny strains of *Für Elise* interrupted our thoughts every now and then.

We worked till the small hours gathering the facts together. These formal comments to the chairman were finished on 28 June. The report which Hempsons had commissioned from Professor Chamberlain some six weeks ago reached us on the 27th. It contained nothing new; if anything, he was less critical of my management of the five cases than I was myself.

Friday, 28 June 1985

We checked our document early on Friday morning and sent it by special messenger to the Regional Legal Adviser at his offices, along with the report from Professor Chamberlain. We both felt pleased. We had finished a mammoth task, it read well, and Brian had given them a deadline of 5 July – or we would go to court. Brian had spoken to John Dennis on the phone and had heard reassuring noises.

This euphoria was wiped out when I returned in the late afternoon. I took one look at Brian's face and knew something was wrong. He handed me Professor Dennis's report – it was terrible. The words 'bizarre and incompetent management', 'consistent aberration of clinical judgement', 'confusing to junior staff and midwives' sprang out of the blurred, old-fashioned type. I turned to the individual case reports. Apart from AU, they were less damning. How had he reached such a devastating conclusion? Had he not done a second report after he had spoken to me and received my draft comments, which filled in the gaps in the case notes?

I felt I had let Brian down by misinterpreting Dennis's friendly behaviour and the, as I thought, frank discussion we had had. Brian had fought so hard for me and he had trusted my judgement. Would he now be wondering if I *was* incompetent? It was one of the worst moments since my suspension. Was I deluding myself? Was Brian's faith in me shattered?

I pulled myself together and apologised to Brian for my misreading of John Dennis. We decided to write a letter to confirm that I did dispute three facts – Trevor Beedham's letter of 21 May 1984, the cause of baby U's death, and the professor's statement that I had failed to make adequate arrangements for my study leave. This was important: if there was no dispute about the facts there need not be an independent enquiry.

It was nearly seven when I left, a hot sticky evening and I had neglected to find myself a partner for the Students' Summer Ball. I rushed home, rang a friend – yes, but no dinner jacket – borrowed one from a neighbour, and we arrived. I had been suspended for nine weeks and two days.

That weekend I showed all the notes, the criticisms and my comments to Professor Ron Taylor and he wrote the following note for Brian:

> I have looked carefully at the five cases which are the subject of
> dispute between Mrs W. Savage and the Tower Hamlets District

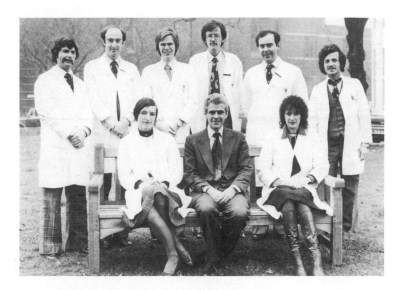

ABOVE
Peter Huntingford,
seated centre; myself,
seated left, and
other members of the
Department of
Obstetrics and
Gynaecology, Mile
End Hospital, 1977

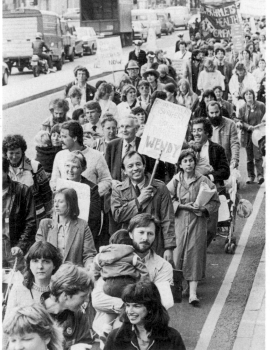

The first march
organised by the
Support Group on 13
July 1985: Tower
Hamlets GPs join with
over 1000 supporters
to demonstrate and
deliver petitions to
Tower Hamlets Health
Authority
(David Hoffman)

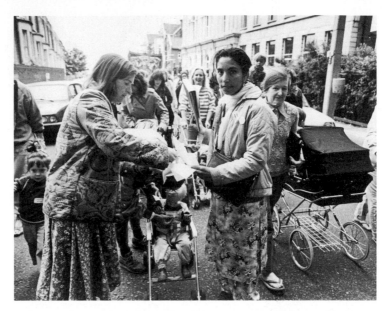

Linda Kaur, whom I've looked after through four pregnancies, collecting signatures for a petition on the march *(David Hoffman)*

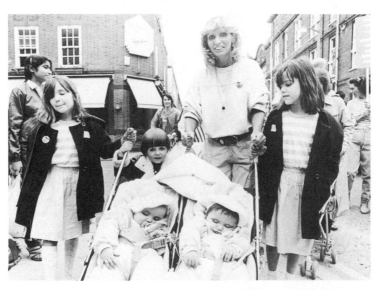

Denise Lewis with her children, expressing her support on the march. Her case was one of the five discussed at the enquiry *(David Hoffman)*

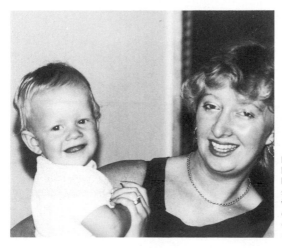

Linda Ganderson with her second baby, born while I was suspended. Her case was one of the five discussed at the enquiry
(Patrick O'Neill)

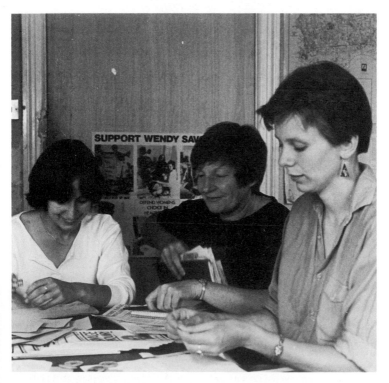

The Wendy Savage Support Campaign in action. From left to right: Heather Reid, Myra Garrett, Sue Hadley *(Ben Thompson)*

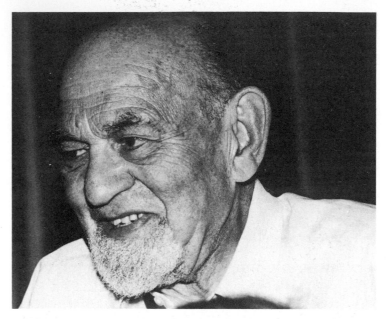

Sam Smith, the Appeal Fund organiser and a great fighter for justice. Sadly he died before the findings of the enquiry were announced *(Ros Reeve)*

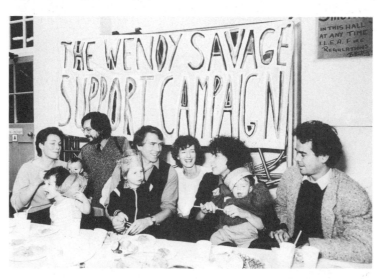

Sitting with Tower Hamlets doctors and families at a children's tea party arranged by the Support Group in January 1986. Tony Jewell and his son Bobby are on my left *(General Practitioner)*

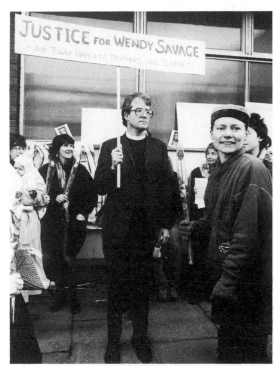

The Support Group
lobbies the enquiry
outside Addison
House. The banner is
held by Richard
Bentley, a local
clergyman *(Ros Reeve)*

BELOW
The panel at the start
of the enquiry. From
left to right:
Mr Leonard Harvey,
Consultant
Obstetrician and
Gynaecologist,
Rugby; Mr
Christopher
Beaumont, the panel's
chairman; Professor
Peter Howie,
Ninewells Hospital,
Dundee
(The Guardian)

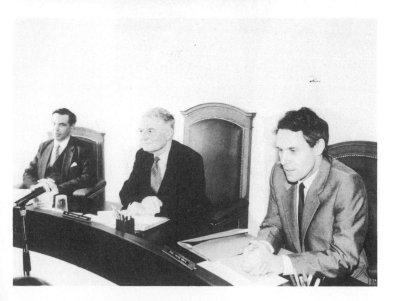

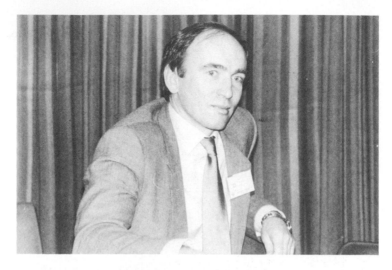

ABOVE
Gedis Grudzinskas,
Professor of
Obstetrics and
Gynaecology at the
London Hospital and
Saint Bartholomew's
Medical Colleges
(The Guardian)

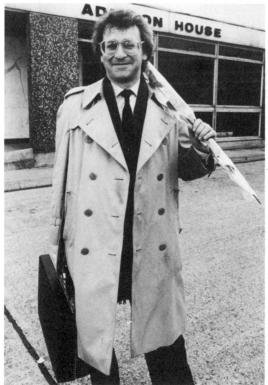

Brian Raymond, my
solicitor, outside
Addison House
(Ros Reeve)

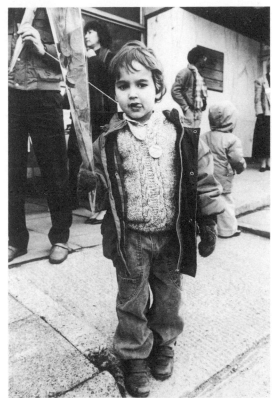

Matthew Reid on the penultimate day of the enquiry after presenting me with a bouquet of flowers
(Ros Reeve)

BELOW
A celebration dinner to mark the end of the enquiry. From left to right: John Hendy, my barrister; Beverley Beech, Chair of the Support Campaign; Brian Raymond, Helena Kennedy, a barrister, who introduced me to Brian, and myself
(Ros Reeve)

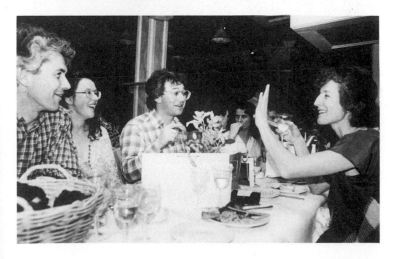

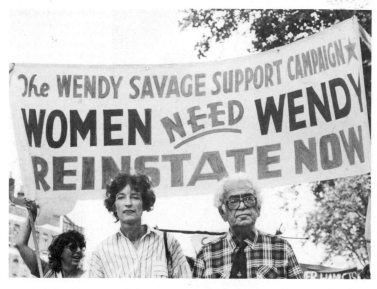

The second march on 10 July 1986 from Mile End to Whitechapel: walking with Ian Mikardo, MP for Bow and Poplar *(Hospital Doctor – photographer: Nick Oakes)*

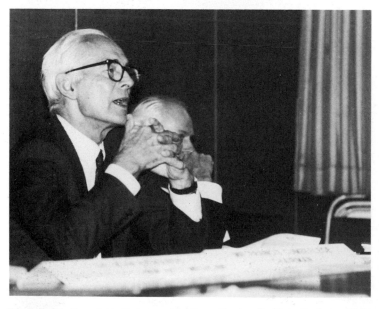

Francis Cumberlege (left), Chairman of the Tower Hamlets Health Authority, and John Alway (right), District General Manager, at the press conference on 24 July 1986 where they announced my reinstatement *(Patrick O'Neill)*

Health Authority. I think that there are matters here where my clinical judgement may have differed from Mrs Savage but in these issues I accept that there is no certain correct management. The issues must be 'was reasonable care exercised' – not 'did the consultant play safe'. We can all play safe to our own advantage and the detriment of the patient. I think very good care was exercised in all these cases – although in two specific incidents, an incorrect decision was made in the absence of the consultant. To my mind there was no question of negligence in any instance . . .

Ron Taylor and I could not be further apart on the issue of abortion, yet his tolerance of my pro-choice stand was in such contrast to the attitudes of some of the other people I knew. It was a relief to hear his judgement. I felt ready to continue the battle.

Tuesday, 2 July 1985

Brian was asked to meet the Deputy Regional Legal Adviser at Addison House, the headquarters of the Regional Legal Office in Chart Street, Islington. After the meeting he called in to my house to tell me the news. The Deputy Legal Adviser had said that there were difficulties with cross-cover between consultants because of our difference in approach. Basically the offer was that if I would go away for six months or so to Oxford or Edinburgh (why not Siberia? I thought), my colleagues, who had been upset by the one-sided publicity, might be able to work with me again. Brian had pointed out that logically that meant that these five cases were not evidence of incompetence or I could hardly come back without having had an enquiry, but the DLA did not want to accept this. He said that if I didn't accept this offer, and suggestions about changing my role to do 'community obstetrics' (i.e. no labour ward work), they would go ahead and have an enquiry. Right at the end, he said this was a 'without prejudice' meeting, that is 'off the record'. I was beginning to understand how the administrative establishment works. This seemed to me to be yet another attempt to get me out of the way now that it was likely that the charge of incompetence would not stick. I told Brian that I was not going to go back as a second-class consultant. If there had to be an enquiry, so be it.

The High Court Action

Our deadline for my reinstatement, 22 July, passed. We had not yet taken counsel's opinion, hoping that it would not be necessary, but Brian rapidly prepared a brief and the following day we met in Old Square, Lincoln's Inn. Upstairs, we each sat at a huge desk, surrounded by bundles of papers tied up in dark pink tape, the bookshelves full of leather-bound tomes. John Hendy, in his late thirties, had been recommended by Brian as an expert in employment law. He said there were three possibilities: defamation, judicial review or breach of contract, and he outlined the pros and cons of each. He thought the third was our best bet, but warned that courts were reluctant to enforce contracts. I felt that he was sizing me up, deciding whether to take the case or not. Suddenly I knew he was going to do it. Rapidly he gave Brian a list of people from whom he would want supporting affidavits, and outlined the way he saw the case being presented.

Our long days and eighty-hour weeks of preparation began again. We began to collect our affidavits. I asked the two vice-presidents of the RCOG and the immediate past-president whether they would swear affidavits. Brian told me titles always went down well with judges but the college was keeping its strictly neutral stance and they all said no.

Monday, 5 August 1985

I went to LBC radio to talk about the issues involved in the case and why we were going to court, and then met Brian and John in Old Square. The Court began at 10 a.m. Outside the Law Courts I greeted the Tower Hamlets women and their babies who had come to support me. We walked in through the back door and found Court 16. The court was crowded. It seemed a pity to be inside this dark, cramped, old-fashioned place, with the barristers in their sombre gear, on such a nice summer day. John Hendy's wig, I noticed, looked a bit untidy, a curl or two loose. I warmed to him for striking a blow for informality. John stood up and explained why we thought an injunction was necessary to force my immediate reinstatement: the loss of service to patients, the damage to me personally, the fact that there were not adequate reasons for my suspension, the long delays common before enquiries under HM(61)112. It sounded convincing to me, but then I was biased.

James Badenoch, representing the DHA, rose next and read the most damaging words from John Dennis and Gordon Bourne. My heart sank. I had thought that once inside a court the full evidence would come out, and the tactic of using selected quotes could no longer be used.

Then John stood up and quoted from Professor Taylor's draft affidavit: 'What is happening to Mrs Savage is not a dispassionate enquiry into her competence but rather a deliberate attempt to manufacture a case against her for the purpose of dismissing her from the staff of the London Hospital Medical College.'

The judge gave the Health Authority two weeks to prepare the case in response to ours, then ten days for us to see their affidavits and prepare our response. We had cleared the first hurdle. I kept calm and tried not to think about the headlines the next day. In fact the press were kind – they picked up the conspiracy theory in the headlines, and quoted Professor Dennis in the body of the text. It could have been much worse.

By 22 August the district had definitely decided to go ahead with a 112 enquiry – and they said it would be held in October. Was it worth going back to court to get my suspension lifted while preparing for the enquiry? We were sceptical about the DHA's date for the enquiry and decided we had nothing to lose.

On 24 August, we received from Mr Dibley the terms of reference for the 112 enquiry which were as follows:

1. In accordance with paragraphs 8 to 15 of circular HM(61)112 to enquire into and report upon the professional competence exhibited by Wendy Diane Savage in her treatment and clinical management of the following cases: Denise Lewis; Susan Payne; Ms X (1986 substitution); Linda Ganderson; AU (1986 substitution).
2. Arising out of the findings and conclusions reached in the enquiry to make such recommendations to the District Health Authority as to any disciplinary action in relation to Wendy Diane Savage as may be deemed appropriate.

What these terms told us was that the enquiry would *not* concern itself with how the case came into being or my overall practice.

So, four and a half months after my suspension, we had a decision about the enquiry. Preparing for the court case had been like working again, even though all those words weren't quite the same as the joy of a delivery, the satisfaction of a well-performed operation, or working out how to help a woman with a sexual problem.

2 September 1985. Return to the High Court

Both my daughters came this time, and the Support Group were there in force. Several women filed into the court, the saris of the Bangladeshi women and the colourful African cloth of the Somali women bringing some colour and life into the place. Once again, the press were overflowing their benches.

This time we made two gains. Firstly, if I was not found to be incompetent I must be reinstated or we could come back to the High Court; and secondly, the judge ruled that the enquiry must take place in a reasonable time.

It soon became clear, however, that even November, the date proposed in the High Court which had influenced the judge's decision not to allow our case to be heard, was not going to be possible, as the members of the panel had not yet been selected.

Going to the High Court had not been a waste of time. Although the affidavits hadn't been read by the judges, they were now available for other people to read. And preparing them had given Brian some idea of the strength of our case.

· CHAPTER 8 ·

The Five Cases

Alas, doctors are judged by their peers not by their patients.

Francis Cumberlege, Chairman of the Tower Hamlets Health Authority

Through all the frustrating months leading up to and during the enquiry, I held on to my conviction that my suspension was *not* about my competence, but was based on an intolerance to a different approach to obstetric care.

Of the five cases, three concerned breech presentation – when the baby is lying bottom, not head, downwards – and one of these women also had twins. Four women were delivered by Caesarean section after labour had been tried, and the fifth had delivered normally, but sadly the baby had died before labour began. Approximately 3 per cent of women will have a breech presentation at term, one in a hundred has twins, and only one woman in a thousand has twin breeches.

In the Mile End branch of the London Hospital the Caesarean section rate, like that in the country as a whole, was about 10 per cent in 1983–4, although in 1984 my personal rate was just over 8 per cent. So clearly these cases had been carefully chosen – 80 per cent of this small group of women had been delivered surgically and 60 per cent had breech presentations!

The Rising Rate of Caesarean Section

In the 1958 national survey done in one week in March, 2.6 per cent of women were delivered by Caesarean section, twice the proportion of those who had this operation in the previous survey at the end of the war in 1946. By the time of the third survey in 1970 the proportion had risen to 4.8 per cent.

Official statistics based on a 10 per cent sample of inpatient records for England and Wales (HIPE), show that the rate continued to rise, to 6 per cent by 1975 and 8.7 per cent by 1980. The 1983 figure for England was 10.1 per cent, and a detailed study in Scotland showed an overall rate of 13 per cent with rates varying from 4.9 per cent to 19.2 per cent in different hospitals in 1982.

Some younger obstetricians speak as if there is no longer any risk to a Caesarean section. It is certainly much lower than ever before, but all surgical operations carry a risk, comparable to those we take willingly every day when we travel by car, cross the road or take part in various sports; Caesarean is no exception. What is clear is that it is safer for the woman to have a vaginal delivery – and moreover she has less 'morbidity', that is infection and haemorrhage and other rarer complications, and she recovers more quickly from a normal birth. After any operation people feel pain in the wound and they feel tired. Looking after a newborn baby, establishing breastfeeding, getting up at night, does not seem the ideal way to recover from surgery.

Although most women cope well with the new baby, more of those delivered by Caesarean section become depressed after they return home, and some studies have shown subtle differences in the ways in which they relate to their babies. In addition, the uterus is scarred, which means a higher chance of an operative delivery next time round, and some work suggests a slightly lower chance of getting pregnant when the woman wants to.

Also, most people think that a Caesarean guarantees a normal healthy baby, but statistically about one and a half to twice as many babies die following a Caesarean operation than if they are delivered head first vaginally. Some of this risk is because the woman may have a complication such as bleeding (ante-partum haemorrhage or high blood pressure), and it is probably in this area that the balance of risk in suggesting one type of delivery over another is most difficult for the obstetrician, with his or her duty to two patients in one body.

The rate of surgical delivery in the USA has risen even faster than on this side of the Atlantic. In 1970 our rates were similar, 4.9 per cent for England and Wales and 5.5 per cent for the USA. By 1983 it was twice as high here, 10.1 per cent, and four times as high, 20.3 per cent, in the States. In 1980 a National Institutes of Health Consensus group – the Task Force – met to discuss the use of Caesarean section in the States, as women and obstetricians were concerned about this rise. They found that breech presentation, repeat Caesarean and 'dystocia' (literally, difficult labour, in practice used loosely to cover 'prolonged' labour, failure to progress, suspected cephalo-pelvic disproportion, etc.) were the most important reasons for the rising rate. The Task Force made several recommendations, including encouraging vaginal birth after previous Caesarean delivery, and allowing vaginal birth for breech babies under 8lbs in weight.

Their recommendations with regard to legal action were:

1. The courts should recognise that if a vaginal birth resulted in a 'less than perfect baby', this does not necessarily mean that the physician was negligent for not performing a Caesarean birth.
2. Physicians should make a determination as to the need for Caesarean section delivery based solely on sound medical judgement.
3. Physicians should support the patient's right to participate in the decision-making process concerning whether to have a Caesarean by proper application of the doctrine of informed consent.

In this country, the legal concept of informed consent is not so strictly drawn, but I have always tried to obtain truly informed consent from a woman by explaining how things are done and why they are necessary.

The Task Force failed in its attempt to halt the steady rise in Caesareans and the provisional figures for 1985 in America are over 24 per cent, almost one woman in four. This is madness. One can only hope that women, midwives and obstetricians will prevent it happening here.

In 1978 the rising rate of Caesarean section at Mile End had caused Peter Huntingford and I to look critically at our practice. When booking a woman for her second or third pregnancy, looking at case notes at the height of the induction era (1974, before Peter had returned to the London) one often saw this sequence of events: induction of labour, often for not very clear reasons, poorly established labour with contractions produced by syntocinon, 'failure to progress', mild fetal distress, 'emergency' Caesarean section – and a healthy non-distressed baby born. Often the conclusion was drawn from this pattern of events that the baby was too big to go through the pelvis (i.e., 'borderline cephalo-pelvic disproportion'), but in the next pregnancy, if allowed to go into labour naturally, four out of five of these women delivered normally – and often the babies were bigger, showing that the suspicion of disproportion was wrong. (Disproportion means that the leading part of the baby is bigger than the bony pelvis and cannot safely be delivered vaginally: if the head is first, then it is called cephalo-pelvic disproportion; when the baby is breech first then it is usually referred to as feto-pelvic disproportion.) I also tried to spend more time in the labour ward with the new registrars, and we arranged some lectures on the interpretation of fetal heart traces (CTGs).

The Caesarean section rate at Mile End, which had risen from 6 to 9.5 per cent between 1975 and 1977, stayed at 9.5 per cent to 10 per cent up to 1984, the last full year I worked before my suspension, but at Whitechapel, where the neonatal intensive care unit is situated, it continued to rise, from 8 per cent in 1976 to 17 per cent in 1985. This may be because more women who are 'at risk' are being referred there, but further analysis needs to be done to establish the reasons for this rise.

Breech Presentation

The question of whether or not women with a breech presentation should be allowed to labour and deliver vaginally or should have a planned Caesarean section – especially if it is a first pregnancy – is one of the most hotly debated topics in obstetrics today.

The evidence about the best way to deliver a baby by the breech is vast, and confusing, and that is why two obstetricians reading the same papers can hold opposing views.

My view is that if the labour goes well in both the first and second stages, and the breech descends on to the perineum naturally, there is no significant risk of the 'obstetrician's nightmare' – that the body of the baby will be delivered and the head becomes stuck above the brim (the top opening) of the pelvis. It was calculated fifty years ago that if the buttocks of the baby would go through the brim of the pelvis then so would a normal-sized head. But it is possible for the head to be held up by an incompletely dilated cervix or if the head is abnormally large, and I think this is where the anxiety stems from.

My own view is that in circumstances where the choices are evenly balanced, the woman's own feelings about the birth should be the deciding factor.

Trial of Labour

If the obstetrician is unsure whether or not the head will pass through the pelvis, a trial of labour is recommended. This means that labour is allowed to progress normally but that preparations are made for a Caesarean section, should this become necessary. In my practice I try to get the same person to do all of the vaginal examinations which tell the doctor how well the labour is progressing.

Sometimes it is necessary to augment labour (strengthen the contractions with syntocinon) to ensure that the woman has had a real 'trial'. Obstetricians also differ about whether or not one can use syntocinon with a scar in the uterus, but my view is that if this is used carefully it is no different from the contractions of normal labour, and one must produce good contractions or the woman will not deliver vaginally. There is no set time for a trial of labour: it depends on the size of the baby and the pelvis, the position of the baby's head and the way that the mother and the baby respond to the labour. As long as there is no maternal or fetal distress I believe that labour can continue although in practice few women are undelivered within twenty-four hours.

Length of Labour

In 1981 I looked at the figures from the hospital computer obstetric databank and found some very interesting differences. My own Caesarean section rate was considerably lower than that of the other consultants: 6.5 per cent compared to a range of 10.9 to 11.9 per cent. This was in part due to the fact that I had more women having their first babies (because I was the newest consultant then) so there were fewer women needing a repeat operation, but in part it seemed to be related to the length of labour. The higher rate at Whitechapel was almost entirely due to the much smaller number of elective Caesarean sections at Mile End (that is, operations planned to be done before labour, compared with emergency sections, which are done once labour has begun or a complication develops).

Of women under my care 12.3 per cent had a labour lasting over twelve hours, compared with between 1.7 per cent and 3.9 per cent under the care of other consultants. It was not that my rate was particularly high – in the 1958 survey a third of women have labours lasting over twelve hours and by 1970 about 20 per cent did so: it was that the others had very low proportions. There was no difference in the percentage of babies needing extra resuscitation at birth or who had low Apgar scores (a measure of the baby's wellbeing at birth).

I looked up the literature about length of labour. I was convinced that one of the reasons for the rising Caesarean section rate was that we were pushing labour on too fast. I went back to the 1958 perinatal mortality survey and here I found some evidence that for women having their first babies, twelve to twenty-four hours labour was associated with the lowest 'mortality ratio'. Why, I wondered, had the survey in 1970 used eighteen hours as the definition of a long labour?

My Obstetric Philosophy

1. Women are different, and each woman and each labour should be managed individually.

2. Midwives and doctors must have clear reasons for procedures and birth management options.

3. Communication between the woman, with or without her partner, and members of the clinical team should be frank and complete.

4. Choice for the woman is important, and midwives and doctors have to overcome their authoritarianism (reinforced by their training) whilst accepting responsibility for life-saving decisions.

In essence these are my ideas on how to approach labour – without rigid rules or routines.

The five cases which Professor Grudzinskas had selected from about 800 women who had had babies under my care during a fourteen-month period in 1983–4 were, as Mr Leigh from Hempsons pointed out to me, 'not my five best cases'. Even so, my policy of having individual plans of management to suit each women had been followed, even if those plans hadn't always been carried out as well as I would have liked. Four of the five cases were very unusual and the fifth, Linda Ganderson, was the only one to have a normal delivery.

When I presented my twenty-two pages of comments on the cases to the Chairman of the Health Authority on 28 June 1985, Brian and I prepared the responses about each case in three parts, the plan of action, where there were departures from ideal management, and my answer to Mr Bourne's specific criticisms.

In July I circulated all members of the Health Authority with the first part of the document and short summaries of each of the cases, which did not reveal the women's identity and which I have used in this chapter.

The criticisms of the professor and Mr Bourne which led the chairman to suspend me have been put separately from those of Professor Dennis, a couple of sentences from his covering letter having been used by the chairman at the July DHA meeting to reinforce the case for the continuation of my suspension.

Professor Chamberlain, affectionately known as 'Bodger' after a rugby player, had been asked by Hempsons to comment on the cases. These reports on the cases were to help the Medical Defence Union advise me to fight or to accept the *prima facie* case of the DHA, and Professor Chamberlain was *not*, as Mr Cumberlege stated, 'the champion selected by Mrs Savage herself'.

The Five Cases

The brief summaries of each case are versions of those I prepared for the Health Authority members in July 1985.

X (initials withheld 1986)
Single. Age 15. 4ft 10 in tall. Delivered 26.9.84.
Trial of labour planned and carried out by my new registrar. Difficulty with the delivery of the baby's head when Caesarean section carried out. Lecturer (honorary senior registrar) called. Next day baby thought by paediatricians to have suffered a fractured skull (extremely rare). Mother and baby well at post-natal examination, done by myself at six weeks.

What were the problems? The baby was lying with its head facing towards the mother's abdomen rather than her back. This happens in 6 per cent of babies coming head first at term, and these labours tend to be longer and more painful.

A trial of labour – one where you are not sure if the baby will be able to pass through the pelvis or not – went well, but at the Caesarean section, it was difficult to deliver the head. This does sometimes happen if the head has been pushed firmly into the pelvis. It requires a knack to release the pressure but this was not an anticipated problem, so I was not there to assist my registrar.

The baby was irritable at birth, which is not uncommon after an eighteen-hour labour and a difficult delivery, and after a skull X-ray, which I did not see at the time, a fracture was diagnosed by the paediatricians caring for the baby.

What went wrong: I should have been there to assist my registrar, so that the anxieties about a possible skull fracture would never have arisen. My registrar had never felt the 'eggshell' sensation of the moulded head where the bones are overlapping one another. Although X and the baby were well at six weeks and the baby has developed normally it was not the best start for a young mother.

Criticisms made before my suspension: Both the professor and Mr Bourne said that the labour lasted too long and said respectively that labour should have ended after twelve or six hours. Mr Bourne thought that the pelvis had not been properly assessed, whereas the professor did not mention this but said that 'it is unfortunate that a more senior person was not present at delivery'.

Comments after my suspension: Professor Dennis said, 'The decision to manage this patient with a trial of labour was justified. The problems occurred at delivery . . .' Professor Chamberlain was sympathetic: 'One can well understand the reluctance of the consultant to do a Caesarean section on a fifteen-year-old girl . . .'

Statements before the enquiry: None of the expert witnesses thought that the management of this young woman's labour could be criticised.

What I think about the case now: Although my registrar did not ask me to assist her, I regret not getting up at 2.45 a.m. as it would probably have made things easier for her and for Ms X but I think it was the right decision to allow her to try and deliver normally. Many of the expert witnesses before the enquiry found great difficulty in understanding why this case had been brought as an example of any shortcomings on my part.

The criticisms were based on a rigid approach to labour, measured in terms of arbitrary timescales rather than observing individual women, and it is this approach that I believe leads to unnecessary Caesarean sections.

AU

Bengali. Age 23. Married. One previous child delivered by Caesarean section. Delivered 26.4.84.

This couple wanted her to try to deliver vaginally and I agreed to a short trial of labour. This commenced on 26.4.84 and AU was delivered that day.

The trial was not conducted as I had outlined. Despite this the baby was delivered in good condition and was noted to be ill forty-eight hours after birth. There was no post-mortem at the parents' request, and I believe the paediatrician's diagnosis can be disputed.

What were the problems? This woman had had a previous operative delivery because of fetal distress after a dysfunctional labour during which the contractions had been augmented with syntocinon. She had not wanted to have a Caesarean but agreed to an operation when advised that the baby was showing signs of distress. However, when the baby was born, he was very active and healthy and her husband who was in the theatre had the opportunity to see that he was not distressed.

When she became pregnant this second time she wanted to deliver vaginally if at all possible. She had a scar in the uterus, and a smaller than average pelvis. It was agreed that she could have a trial of labour and then the baby turned to be a breech. (Breech babies have less time for the head to mould as it goes through the pelvis and so a baby, who could be delivered head first, may not go through in the breech position, even though it is the same size.) Then her labour was dysfunctional again, which might have been because the baby was too big (although that is not as likely a cause in a second pregnancy as in a first), but it needed augmentation if we were going to let her have a proper trial of labour.

What went wrong: I was not aware of the opposition of the lecturer to allowing this woman to experience a trial of labour, which led to some difficulties in communication. This meant that the labour lasted longer than I had planned.

The critics' response: Mr Bourne had a list of nine criticisms which can be summarised as:
– trial of labour is contra-indicated if the pelvic inlet is less than 10cm (the normal range is 10–14cm with an average of about 11.5 in British women).
– if the baby is presenting by the breech, syntocinon should not be given.

Mr Bourne and the professor would have done an elective Caesarean section, as I would have if the woman had not wanted to do otherwise. Mr Bourne said, 'This patient was not managed by normal standard practice and a disastrous outcome was almost certainly inevitable.' But he did not commit himself to saying why the baby died.

Professor Dennis said that the woman would 'almost certainly have agreed' to an elective section – but of course he had not spoken to her! He considered that my management was 'bizarre and incompetent' (a phrase that Mr Cumberlege read out in the July DHA meeting).

Professor Grudzinskas stated that the cause of death was thought to be a tentorial tear leading to intracerebral bleeding, but Professor Dennis considered that the baby died 'from anoxia caused by strong uterine contractions affecting the placental circulation in the presence of disproportion'. Professor Chamberlain, who did not have the criticisms of this case sent to him, speculated that 'the ultimate bad outcome may have been related to hypoxia in labour'.

Anoxia means no oxygen and hypoxia means a shortage of oxygen, but in my experience, if a baby has been starved of oxygen for a damaging period during labour or delivery it has fits soon after birth because of the damage to the most sensitive tissues in the body, the brain cells. This new theory of the cause of the baby's death was to be a major focus for Mr Kennedy's cross-examination during the enquiry, but had not been a criticism in the original *prima facie* case against me.

What I feel about the U case now: I regret that I did not understand how opposed the lecturer was to allowing the woman to experience labour, even though I knew that the chance of her delivering vaginally was remote. Had I done so, I would have taken over the case completely in the morning.

The principle that a woman should be able to have a trial of labour, even if I do not think she will succeed, as long as she and the baby are all right, is one that I stand by, but I wish I had spent longer explaining the situation myself to the couple.

I also feel deeply saddened by the way the enquiry into my competence has affected the Us and their ability to mourn for their baby in privacy, and with the understanding of their own doctor.

One of the worst moments of the last fifteen months has been the sight of Mrs U on television saying that she had trusted me, and my awareness that she thought I had let her down.

Denise Lewis
English. Married. Age 26. Twins 1976, 8lb 1oz baby 1980. Delivered 5.7.84.
Breech presentation of both twins, raised blood pressure and anaemia. The major criticism was of the management of labour which was conducted by the lecturer and my registrar when I was on study leave. The professor was asked for his advice about this woman at 3 p.m., ordered no specific treatment, and did not see her until 7.50 p.m. Caesarean section was performed at 9.20 p.m. and resulted in the delivery of two live, healthy children. The mother also did well. I had made adequate arrangements for my cover whilst on leave.

What were the problems? Denise developed anaemia, which did not respond to the usual treatment with pills and then injections. She later received a blood transfusion for this. She also developed high blood pressure at the end of her pregnancy, and as soon as this happened I arranged for her labour to be started off, in case of any risk of eclampsia (fits). The syntocinon drip which was used to do this did not work. I was on study leave but in order to minimise the burden on David Oram, the consultant who was 'covering' my cases, I came into the hospital at the beginning and end of each day.

What went wrong? Medically speaking, nothing went wrong but communication was not good. The message that I gave to my SHO to give to the lecturer was apparently not clear enough for him to understand. When my registrar took over at lunchtime he and the lecturer did not speak directly to each other, so the registrar was unclear about the plan of management. He then rang the professor who was the duty consultant but was not standing in for me during my study leave.

Criticisms made before my suspension: The anaemia had not been investigated adequately, or treated properly. They said she had had severe pre-eclampsia in June (which was not correct), and that she should have been delivered by elective rather than emergency (done after a trial of labour) Caesarean section. My plan of management was 'insufficiently defined' and my arrangements for study leave were criticised.

Comments after my suspension: Professor Dennis thought that her 'problems were not treated with adequate urgency and I must judge the patient fortunate not to have suffered more severe complications'.

Professor Chamberlain said he would need more information before commenting on the administrative matters and as far as elective Caesarean section was concerned, 'It might be expected that labour would proceed apace and Mrs Savage's view could probably be defended.'

Comments made at the enquiry by expert witnesses: Gordon Stirrat's reply to the question of any incompetence on my part in this case was: 'In no way, shape or form can Mrs Savage's management be described as incompetent in this regard. If it were I would suggest that the majority of obstetricians in this country are similarly incompetent.'

What Denise thought: Denise, who has been one of my most stalwart supporters, appeared with her two sets of twins and her daughter at meetings and demonstrations, and offered to give evidence at the enquiry. She did not want to have a Caesarean, and was glad to have had an opportunity to try to deliver normally. She had nothing but praise for her care.

What I think now: I should have spoken directly to the lecturer so that no confusion could have arisen.

Susan Payne

English. Married. Age 24. First baby. 6ft 1in tall. Delivered 5.8.83. Breech presentation: for planned vaginal delivery. The second stage lasted longer than usual, and although it is not my usual practice, I used syntocinon to see if vaginal delivery could be achieved, as the baby was not large (6lbs 13oz). There were problems with communication, but I assisted my new registrar with the Caesarean section and mother and baby were well. She has since delivered a 7lbs 11oz baby vaginally after a 2½ hour labour, under my care.

What was the problem? After normal first stage of labour lasting about twelve hours, the cervix was fully dilated but the labour virtually stopped. Because this was so unusual, I thought it might be because she had had an epidural (a pain-relieving injection of anaesthetic round the spinal cord) which had then been repeated twice, so I thought we should wait for this to wear off as both mother and baby were well.

I expected the contractions to return, but they did not, and having checked personally the size of the baby and the bony pelvis, I thought we would augment labour with syntocinon. The baby had still, inexplicably, failed to descend into the pelvis, so she had a Caesarean section, with which I helped my registrar.

What went wrong? I should have gone to assess things as soon as my registrar telephoned me, which would have saved some time. However, the mother and baby were well and this did not affect the outcome.

Criticisms before my suspension: Professor Grudzinskas and Mr Bourne said I should have done a Caesarean section as soon as the second stage – defined as the time when the cervix becomes fully dilated – was prolonged, and that I should not have used syntocinon to strengthen the contractions with a breech presentation. Interestingly, in his draft reports Mr Bourne said: the use of syntocinon is 'totally and completely' contra-indicated and there was a third paragraph which read: 'It is possible and highly probable that this patient survived only because this was her first child. Had this been anything other than her first child then it would seem reasonable to suggest that because of this delay her uterus would have ruptured and a disastrous situation would have followed.'

Uterine rupture in a woman having her first baby is exceedingly rare – and as the reason that Susan's labour was not progressing was because her contractions had virtually stopped, this risk was a non-starter.

Criticisms after my suspension: Professor Chamberlain found this 'the most difficult case to defend, for eight hours in the second stage in a breech presentation is well outside the normal range of behaviour', whereas Professor Dennis described my management as 'eccentric'. At the enquiry these criticisms were changed halfway through my cross-examination after John Hendy had exposed the weakness of the case.

Comments before the enquiry: John McGarry had this to say: 'This, however, is a highly unusual case and I do not believe that Mrs Savage's management can be faulted. It seems extremely curious to me that this case is used as an example of poor management on Mrs Savage's part', and he suggested that it should have been written up 'for a scientific journal as an example of a wholly inexplicable occurrence, namely the failure of the breech to descend and pass normally through what must be regarded as a gigantic pelvis.'

What Susan thought about her care: Susan was very satisfied with her care, otherwise, as she pointed out, she wouldn't have chosen me again as her consultant. On TV later she said, 'When I heard that she had been accused and my baby's birth was being used against her, I just left the children and went into the kitchen and had a good swear – even my husband said, "It can't be possible." '

Linda Ganderson
English. Married. Age 27. First baby. Delivered 22.4.84.
The baby did not grow well, this was recognised by the GP when I was on holiday. The woman was admitted to hospital for investigation, allowed home for Easter, and came back with a small amount

of bleeding. Immediate action was not taken and the baby died undelivered the next day. Since then she became pregnant again and has safely delivered. Despite careful monitoring, growth retardation again occurred late, her GP alerted the hospital and Trevor Beedham induced her labour and all was well.

What were the problems? At thirty-two weeks the uterus was noted to be small. Was this because the baby was not growing well or because she conceived after her monthly egg had been produced late? When it was decided that the baby was not growing well some weeks later, she then had a small amount of bleeding. The question was, should her labour have been induced then?

What went wrong? Due to an administrative error I did not see Linda at thirty-six weeks when I had planned and this meant that I was on holiday when a week later her GP correctly made the diagnosis of intrauterine growth retardation (IUGR).

When admitted to hospital no consultant opinion was obtained, and with hindsight one could see that the significance of the baby's growth retardation was not appreciated.

Criticisms before my suspension: Mr Bourne had seven paragraphs on this case and said that, 'Obviously this patient was mismanaged, but the apportionment of blame is difficult because everybody began to assume that the intrauterine growth retardation was caused by "wrong dates".' He, like the other commentators, John Dennis and Bodger Chamberlain, did not know that I was on holiday when Linda was admitted.

I had had considerable correspondence with Gedis about this case and had sent him a case report so he could answer the 'gossip' he said had occurred after the May 1985 perinatal mortality meeting. He agreed with Mr Bourne that shared care should have ended as soon as growth retardation was even suspected, and said she should have been classified to 'full consultant care' and that her delivery should have been earlier. He *did* know that I was on holiday.

Criticisms after my suspension: John Dennis said, 'The diagnosis of intrauterine growth retardation was made in good time. The action taken as a result seems to be sluggish. The infant died in utero as a result of an error of judgement. Such an error can occur in the experience of any obstetrician on an occasional basis.'

Comments made by experts before the enquiry: Professor Taylor said that, 'I cannot accept that admitting this woman at thirty or thirty-two weeks would have been a sensible way to proceed.' Edmund Hey said, 'I find it difficult to see what objective grounds we have for faulting management until thirty-four weeks after the last menstrual period and Mrs Savage has already conceded that an error of management occurred at that time.' John McGarry: 'I cannot see any reason why this woman should not have received shared care.'

What I think about Linda Ganderson now: One of the most difficult situations for any doctor is explaining to a patient that something was not done perfectly – especially if the end result is bad. Nobody is perfect and mistakes do occur, so all mature doctors will have had to face the fact that their good intentions have sometimes resulted in harm – sometimes even death. In obstetrics, maternal deaths are now rare, and the average obstetrician qualified in the last ten years will not have more than two or three women under his or her care die in a lifetime. However, one baby in every hundred dies inside the uterus or in the first week of life so most obstetricians will have between five and ten women a year who leave hospital without a live baby. In about a quarter or a third of these women, a different course of action would probably have saved the baby's life. As an obstetrician one's own feelings of guilt in this situation can be overwhelming, and the doctors must be honest, with themselves primarily, before they can discuss things honestly with the parents.

One of the most difficult tasks is to ensure that one deals with the parents' feelings of grief, whilst admitting to one's own errors in such a way that the trust between the parents and the doctor is not destroyed. One must not unload guilt to make oneself feel better but the parents worse. The most difficult situation for me is trying to be honest with the parents whilst not criticising actions of the junior staff who, because of their inexperience, may have missed something which I probably would have seen. As a consultant, the responsibility for the work carried out by junior staff is yours – though one cannot be in the hospital twenty-four hours a day, fifty-two weeks a year. I try to do ward rounds or visit the antenatal wards every day, to be at the end of a bleep or a telephone, and to create a climate in which they feel free to discuss potential problems as well as situations which need an immediate decision.

When I returned from my holiday and was told of Linda Ganderson's stillbirth I felt responsible – not because I had delegated care to the GP for which I was so heavily criticised by the professor, Gordon Bourne and John Dennis – but because I had not been there when the GP picked up the IUGR, and not there for my registrar or the senior registrar to consult when she was admitted. I explained to Linda that probably there had been a further amount of bleeding on the morning the baby had died which had been the last straw as the baby had not been growing well for some time.

I have Linda's permission to use her case, and she has seen successive drafts as I have written them. For her the publicity of the enquiry was painful and opened old wounds, but I hope that by sharing her experience with other women – and doctors – we will all learn to the benefit of women in the future.

· CHAPTER 9 ·

The Run-Up to the Enquiry

The law is not about justice; and justice is expensive.

Brian Raymond

Preparing the Defence

We had agreed with Mr Dibley that Brian and I would prepare the typewritten transcript of the case notes to be used in the enquiry. The first task was to get the various missing parts of the case notes, the CTG's, the X-rays of the mothers and babies, and the ultrasound scan for Baby U from the hospital records department. We also needed to track down the notes of Baby X which had never been sent to us; I had done my comments for the chairman of the Health Authority from the mother's notes. We wrote off for these and then began to go through the material with a fine tooth comb.

I knew that a baby of 2.9 kg with a normal sized head could be safely delivered through a pelvis with an inlet of 9.5 cm because of my experience in Africa. I spent some time in the library checking these references.

We had still not received all the notes, and as we were going through them I noticed other omissions: the treatment sheet and some of the nursing notes in the U case, the first EEG report on baby U, the pre-eclampsic toxaemia (PET) charts on Denise Lewis, the labour CTG on Ms X, one of Susan Payne's X-rays, some laboratory forms. By mid October we still had not received the ultrasound scans of Baby U, and I learnt that they had been sent to Mr Dibley without copies having been made for us. I rang him myself – and he told me that to do so was quite improper, I had to communicate via my solicitor. Such strict protocol seemed very strange to me. I needed them urgently because I had asked Sid Watkins to look at the notes and scan with his neurosurgical eye, and he was going away. So, finally I went to Addison House where

100

Mr Dibley worked, and demanded to see him. When he came down to the lobby with a photocopy, which was not adequate for our purposes, I said I had to have the copy film by nine the next morning. I offered to take it and have it copied myself. He was horrified at the very thought. But if he was adamant, so was I, and I got the film the next morning in time to give to Sid.

On 3 December Mr Dibley sent us the full list of charges (see Appendix I). Now we were able to start the detailed rebuttal of these fifty-nine items. As we finished each case, these responses and the annotations were sent to brief our counsel. By the second week in December we still did not have Baby X's notes along with the other details we had requested, so I asked Brian to ask Mr Dibley if I could go to his office and search for the missing items from the original notes. This time he agreed, and twice that week I spent five hours going through the notes and listing what was needed, including copies of the CTG traces.

I collected Baby X's films from the hospital a fortnight later. I had never seen these X-rays before. Two radiologists were in the room. I took them out of the packet and looked at them carefully. I could not see any skull fracture. I passed them to one of the two radiologists. He looked at them in silence and passed them to the second who scanned them both. 'Who reported on these?' he said. I read out the registrar's name. They looked at each other and said nothing. I knew I was right – there was no fracture. This was confirmed by the expert paediatricians when I sent the copies to them.

Brian's secretary, Hilary, was snowed under with annotations and my lengthy comments. Over Christmas and the New Year, with all the information together at last, both Brian and I and a temporary secretary worked for hours on the transcripts, checking them against notes. It seemed endless.

The starting date of the enquiry was Monday 3 February 1986. It struck me that if a woman had her last menstrual period on the 24 April 1985, the day I was suspended, her estimated date of delivery would be the first of February. The third was the first working day after this. It seemed fitting somehow that a case centred on obstetrics should have this kind of time scale. By the time the enquiry was over the pregnancy was well beyond term!

The Selection of the Expert Witnesses

Although an enquiry panel is set up to look into the accused doctor's competence, there was no doubt that this one was going to be, in effect, a trial, and its adversarial nature was made very clear on 1 December when we received the list of the prosecution's witnesses (and their statements): my four consultant colleagues, the lecturer and one of the senior registrars involved in Linda Ganderson's case, one registrar and two senior house officers. The junior staff had written statements about their personal involvement in the cases, but my colleagues had also put in their own opinions, criticising my management in strong terms. We wondered who their expert witnesses were going to be. Even at this point I thought John Dennis might refuse. After all, he had done his report very quickly, in one day, and at the time he lacked all the documentation. I had been told that he had not given his permission for his reports to be read out in the High Court.

I also wondered if Gordon Bourne would appear. Professor Taylor had given evidence in his affidavit that Bourne's report did not constitute 'any form of external scrutiny in that he was closely associated with Professor Grudzinskas when the latter worked under him at St Bartholomew's Hospital'. Peter Huntingford's affidavit had recounted how Gordon Bourne had opposed my appointment at the London and he, in turn, denied this in his own affidavit. However, just before Christmas we had heard that Bourne and Dennis were to be the Health Authority's expert witnesses.

I found the whole question of involving junior staff as witnesses for my defence difficult, fearing that their support for me could damage their careers. I deliberately chose to ask those of my staff who were not planning to continue a career in obstetrics, except for one who particularly wanted to give evidence in my defence because of her commitment to women and to feminism. She was in a good training scheme so I did not think her support of me would damage her. When I was preparing my case for the High Court I had asked two of my registrars for affidavits. One was doing venereology and one was a principal in general practice. Katie Simmons had done a locum registrar post for me, had worked for Peter Huntingford and had also finally decided to do general practice. The SHOs I asked were now all doing general practice.

What we needed were expert witnesses to discuss the disputed points of management. We decided not to use all the people we had asked to give affidavits, partly to keep the opposition guessing and partly because we were now looking at the details of the five cases, whereas in the summer when we went to the High Court we had been arguing that my suspension was unjustified. For the first time we had an advantage; instead of responding to other people's initiatives, we did not have to reveal our witnesses until the case started.

Ron Taylor's understanding of my approach, combined with his own wide clinical experience and knowledge of community ante-natal care, made him an essential expert witness. He was also a man of principle: I thought that this attribute was the most important. People might have different ideas about the best clinical management, but those with principles would accept that in most cases in medicine there are different approaches to the same problem and would understand my viewpoint – even if they themselves would do things differently.

Rather than calling only London obstetricians, whose day-to-day contacts with my colleagues might become an embarrassment, I thought it would be better to call medical witnesses from different parts of the country. I also thought this would broaden the debate. As far as the paediatricians were concerned, I asked Peter Dunn, Reader at Bristol, whom I had heard speak a couple of times; he was also President of the British Perinatal Paediatric Group. On the advice of a colleague of Sid Watkins, I got in touch with Edmund Hey, whom I had never met. And through Carole Desateux, a paediatric senior registrar at Great Ormond Street who had her baby under my care and whose partner works as a GP in the South Poplar Health Centre, I approached Professor Campbell in Aberdeen. I had never met him either.

John McGarry from Barnstaple, whom I knew through Doctors for a Woman's Choice on Abortion, was one of the obstetricians I asked. Another, James McGarry, I had heard speak thoughtfully about Caesarean section at a conference. From Glasgow, he had worked in Nairobi before I was there. Glasgow University had a link in Nairobi, and I always felt that my most important formal obstetrics training had been Glaswegian even though it had occurred in Africa. I wanted a woman, and Marion Hall from Aberdeen, whom I knew slightly, had done a lot of work on antenatal care. Again I knew nothing of her practice, except that, on the whole, Scottish obstetricians spent more time in the labour ward than their London counterparts. Iain Chalmers, who runs the National Perinatal Epidemiology Unit, I had met through work; we were both members of the Forum of Obstetrics and the Newborn. I chose him because I wanted an obstetric epidemiologist to put the range of opinions into a scientific framework – and to comment on the validity of the selection of five cases as a way of assessing competence. Gordon Stirrat, Professor at Bristol, I did not know personally and I knew nothing about his research interests or obstetric practice, but I knew he was a Christian and opposed to abortion. When we met in Brian's office soon before Christmas I found him impressive and intelligent.

Along with the letters going to and from the witnesses, I sent them case notes, affidavits, and copy X-rays. Hilary and I worked till 5 p.m. on Monday 23 December making sure that the last of these parcels, containing the photocopied CTGs, and the missing bits of notes received from Mr Dibley, got there in time for our experts to use the Christmas break to study them.

In the new year Brian Raymond embarked upon a tour of the country, going to Glasgow, Aberdeen, Bristol and Barnstaple to collect the statements from our experts in relation to the specific charges – a massive task, but he returned from these expeditions more and more cheerful as he realised what a strong case we had.

I spent many hours going through the transcribed notes, line by line, with John Hendy. Every day I drove down to Lincoln's Inn with large files, references, books and papers. I had borrowed one of the bony pelvises and dolls we used for teaching, and I showed John the mechanics of breech delivery and the difference between a footling and a complete breech and a frank breech. One day we went to Queen Charlotte's and the radiologist explained to him all the features of the pelvimetry and the ultrasound films that we had. I was amazed at the way all this information was absorbed and how he could find his way through the mass of papers.

We finished our preparation by Friday, 31 January. There was nothing more that we could do. The transcripts had been checked by the Health Authority, amended, interleaved with photocopied notes and put into different coloured folders. Large cardboard boxes were used to transport them to Addison House where the enquiry was to take place.

A friend of mine had bought me a respectable suit in a Jaeger sale, and on the Saturday I went out to buy a blouse. I returned some hours later with several blouses, shoes, matching handbags, a leather jacket, a bookcase and an Amstrad computer. As my youngest son unloaded the car, he looked in disbelief, 'I thought you went out to buy a blouse, not the whole of London.' The day before the enquiry we unpacked the Amstrad, attempted to understand the manual and assembled the bookcase so that I had somewhere other than the floor of my study to put all the reference material overflowing from my bookshelves. I had only just taken down my Christmas cards and needed the string in the hall to put up all the cards that had been arriving to wish me good luck.

That night I slept well: a medical training prepares you as well as most for this kind of situation. We had done the work, now the exam was ahead and we would either pass or fail.

· CHAPTER 10 ·

The Enquiry Begins

Who shall decide when doctors disagree.

Alexander Pope, *Moral Essays*

The Prosecution Case

On Monday 3 February I woke at 6 a.m. and left the house in the
dark. Brian had arranged for me to do BBC Breakfast Time as well
as TV AM, which had been booked for weeks, followed by LBC
in Gough Square before getting to Addison House. He arrived to
collect me in the taxi, and we drove to Lime Grove. Denise Lewis
and her incredibly placid eighteen-month-old twins were also on
the programme, quite relaxed in front of the lights, and the short
interview went well.

The next interview was more difficult – I was asked if I thought
all this would have happened to a man, and I really had not thought
about that for ages; I answered as best I could but I didn't feel
that I had done it well. LBC, on the other hand, was much more
relaxed. I decided again that I much prefer doing radio to TV and
it doesn't take half as much time. As we left another radio reporter was there with his machine, and then we were arriving at
Addison House.

It was a cold grey morning, but already at 9.30 there were
dozens of women and their babies outside, plus press photographers and TV cameras. Heather Reid's son, Matthew, gave me
a bunch of flowers from the Support Group, I posed for photographs with Carol Lefevre and her twins, seeing all the familiar
faces of women I had cared for and those who had fought for me
over the last ten months – Sue, Myra, Beverley, the MSLS
workers. A clergyman carried a banner saying 'Justice for Wendy
Savage'; I hoped he would be proved right. Clutching two large
ring-binders, a large bouquet of flowers, a bunch of freesias and

106

cards from well-wishers, I went through the door into the foyer where we were greeted by the woman in charge of the arrangements and shown to our room – about ten feet square, windowless, cream paint stripped off where sellotaped notices had been removed, a cardboard-wrapped filing cabinet and two desks, and the boxes from Bindmans with all the case notes in folders, the affidavits, the pelvis and doll. This was to be our base for the next five weeks. I met our clerk, Phil, a medical student having a year off. John arrived and we moved the furniture around, got permission to use the new filing cabinet, and checked out the phone. Then it was time to start, so down the corridor past the security guards. I didn't wear my badge – I assumed they would know who I was!

The room where we were to sit was the Council Chamber where the Area Health Authority had held their meetings. Today as we entered, I saw that the opposition were on the left; the middle tier of three rows was packed with the press, and we were to sit at the front on the right. Phil sat behind with the tape-recorder and our supporters, almost all women, sat in the top third row. As we sat down, I studied the other side: Mr Ian Kennedy QC, glasses, slightly receding dark hair, mid-fifties, a little overweight, setting up a folding lectern for himself. Next to him in the front row, James Badenoch, who had represented the THHA in the High Court, fairer, younger, a more open face, turning to talk to Gedis Grudzinskas, sitting in the second row. On his left a very heavy-set, middle-aged man and next to him another slighter, more dapper lawyer with a watch chain across his waistcoat. On the professor's left sat Mr Dibley, his bushy eyebrows twitching as he rustled the papers anxiously, and then a smaller man with a goatee. And in the back row, a very neat, young, dark-haired man, their law clerk. The contrast between this phalanx of sober-suited men with their often loud middle-class voices and the less formally dressed women on our side, with John Hendy, tall 'as a beanpole' as Jeremy Laurence from *New Society* put it, and Brian and myself in the front row, reflected the battle of a group of establishment men versus a somewhat non-conformist woman.

The door on the opposite side of the room opened and in came the panel – we all stood up just as we had in the High Court. The panel, set up by the Joint Consultants Committee of the BMA, comprised Leonard Harvey, the BMA nominee, Consultant in Obstetrics and Gynaecology from Rugby; Christopher Beaumont, the chairman, a barrister chosen from the panel maintained by the DHSS, and Peter Howie, the RCOG nominee, Professor of Obstetrics and Gynaecology in Dundee. Len Harvey I'd met once – he came and sat nearest to us; the chairman was obviously the tall, white-haired man who took the middle chair, and Peter Howie, the Scottish professor, sat farthest away from us on Beaumont's left. Cameras flashed as the panel, ourselves and the other side were photographed. Then everything settled down and at about 11.15 Mr Beaumont opened the proceedings: the timing of the meetings, the request for tape-recording the proceedings so that Claire Dyer of the *BMJ* could do weekly reports and Mr Kennedy's grudging acceptance. Then lunch and tea arrangements – it seemed we would never get down to the case itself. Sitting at a little table between the lawyers in front of Mr Beaumont and facing us was the shorthand writer, writing rapidly. In the space between the seats was a larger table on which were piled the five ring-binders containing the case notes. Brian, referred to formally by John as 'my instructing solicitor', handed duplicate sets of these to the panel members. They did not have enough room on their curved table for everything so some went on the floor.

The chairman referred to 'Mrs Savage being the only one on trial' when the lawyer with the watch chain identified himself as Mr Conlin from the Medical Protection Society, there to represent the interests of all the London Hospital doctors. The chairman then mentioned that this was somewhere between an enquiry and an adversarial system. When he ruled that the women would be referred to by their initials, Mr Kennedy pointed out that that would not be sufficient 'cloak' because of the publicity, and John Hendy told the chairman that we had permission from Mrs P., Mrs G., and Mrs L. to use their names publicly, but not the others. Mr Kennedy introduced the 'compendium' of all the criticisms and my comments in a sixty-nine-page 'bundle', and the documents relating to my appointment, including the 1977 curriculum vitae (CV). John Hendy said he thought my up-to-date CV was more relevant, and casually mentioned that we were proposing to put that in with the affidavits which had made up our case to the High Court. I waited for the chairman to say that they were irrelevant, but he said nothing, and neither did the other side. Finally Mr Kennedy got to his feet.

I could hardly believe my ears as he started off with a long speech about what this case was *not* about – *not a contest between the old and new, or between technology and the woman's freedom to choose how, when and where to have their babies.* He must have been reading the press cuttings: *my colleagues in no way criticise or do not subscribe to many of the philosophies that Mrs Savage supports.* Good news – so when they are reassured about my competence we'll all be able to work together again seemed the logical extension of that line of argument. *The question is not about the principle. The question is about the way that it was put into practice in these five individual cases, and it is an enquiry not into theories, but about dangers in obstetrics.*

Here we go again, I thought: the same argument put forward by the professor to convince the DHA that obstetrics should be centralised at Whitechapel. The barrister will put forward the views of his client, transformed into legal language, but that is in essence his job, to make the best case, however poor the material. *Of the five cases, one resulted in neonatal death and another in a stillbirth. One does not like to have to advance these matters in a public debate, but since it has to be in public it has to be in public, but one must say that the evidence we would call will suggest that both these sadnesses could and should have been avoided. In the remaining cases the management was outside all normally accepted principles and exposed the mothers and their babies to risks which were both real and not necessary.* I looked at the press scribbling away furiously – it sounded very convincing. To me it was not new. Would Andy Veitch, who had covered the case so well in the *Guardian* since the beginning, wonder if he had made a mistake? *The answer has been made in a number of instances that no harm was done and this has been relied upon as justification of the judgement at the time, but we must remind ourselves that this is also the answer of the driver who rounds a blind corner on the wrong side of the road* . . . He went on in the same vein – one hour to get a Caesarean at Mile End so must tailor practice . . . confusing junior staff . . . plans inadequate . . . I should have been there . . . I was critical of junior staff . . . perinatal death led to a complaint . . . other cases came to light because of the concern of my colleagues and junior staff . . . end of preliminary remarks. Now I thought he would list the charges, maybe not all fifty-nine, but suitably shortened. However, he did not.

Instead he began to go slowly through the case notes, almost as if he was reading them for the first time. He began with Susan Payne. Suddenly Professor Howie leant forward and in his quiet, accented voice he said, *There is a technical confusion. At one point it says that there is a footling presentation and at another point it says it's a complete breech. These two are mutually exclusive and that is a matter of considerable obstetric importance.* Kennedy turned to Professor Grudzinskas and after a whispered discussion said that it was not clear what the presentation was. My spirits rose; obviously Peter Howie was not going to allow sloppiness. Gedis had incorrectly described the presentation in his summary and Gordon Bourne and John Dennis had accepted this. Peter Howie asked for the X-rays. They were not forthcoming. Kennedy looked irritated: *your point will be attended to.* He continued his slow progress through the notes. I began to see how they had thought we needed four weeks. He came to a *notation in the left hand margin.* John Hendy rose to his feet: *it was the professor's telephone number at Whitechapel where Mrs Savage was going.* Suddenly the scene sprang to life – it was not all paper and words – a ripple of laughter ran round the room.

Mr Kennedy continued on through the notes and then summarised the criticisms. Professor Dennis said I should have been there all the time; Gordon Bourne said there was *no reason why the section should have been delayed for so long.* I'd explained in June 1985 how it happened. Then Kennedy read out the whole of Professor Chamberlain's comments on this case – naturally – as Bodger had found it the most difficult to defend and had thought that I had not come in to do the operation, which I had. Mr Kennedy could have seen that in the typewritten transcript, even if he couldn't read my registrar's handwriting in the notes. Gedis could have told him, had they sat down and gone through the notes as John and I had. John Hendy corrected the error, *Thank you. I do not know how he came to make the mistake, but there it is,* said Kennedy.

He turned to Linda Ganderson, and Professor Howie showed that he had read the notes as he directed Mr Kennedy to the redrawn antenatal page which we were all to have indelibly imprinted on our memories by the time the case was finished. Several times John Hendy drew his 'learned friend's' attention to errors as he went through the notes. I had not been prepared for the pauses: the turning over of pages of the notes to find the evidence, the picking up and slowly finding the place in the compendium. I realised that my idea of court procedure was heavily influenced by films and plays in which the drama, not the tedium, comes over. Kennedy criticised me for not intervening earlier. John asked him to read the part of my comments where I explained I was on holiday, thus destroying his argument. But Kennedy raised the question of the 'uncertainties of the junior staff'. It was lunchtime.

I realised that my period had started – I hadn't had one for three months and thought I'd reached the menopause, glad that it seemed I was to be part of that 20 per cent of women who don't have symptoms like hot flushes. I looked in my new handbag, I had not put in any tampons. Somehow it seemed symbolic – men never had to think about such things interrupting their lives. There was no handy chemist and the tight skirt and high heels I was wearing made it impractical to nip out to Old Street and look for one. I spoke to the woman in charge and she found some for me. We smiled at each other as I disappeared into the toilet.

We took the lift to the top floor, queued behind the opposition in the canteen and then watched them enter the 'directors' dining room', a little closed-off, glassed-in room up two steps, opening on to a roof garden. We had a screened-off area at the other end of the canteen – the food was plentiful, rather like school and provided free; the women serving were very cheerful and everybody was very nice to us. We reviewed the morning – no worse than expected – I understood the meaning of the phrase 'he hadn't read his brief'.

Then back to the chamber where the windows are covered by long, thick curtains kept drawn, and the ceiling curves up into a strange inverse turret of wood and dark glass. With the soft carpet, the subdued lighting and the closed curtains, it was like going into a space capsule, and as the day went on the feeling of unreality became stronger. That afternoon Kennedy made several errors as he went through AU's notes – as well as making his position clear when reading out my explanation as to why I had allowed a trial of labour: *if a repeat Caesarean was deemed necessary she would feel that she had had a chance to deliver normally. Again, with respect* – I understood that whenever a particularly telling point is being made the lawyers drew attention to it by saying 'with respect', as Kennedy did now – *a slightly remarkable statement because most women would be prepared to accept the advice of their consultant.* I felt that was his own view of the world. He stressed that my management was likely to result in severe damage or death, but only when he came to the fourth case, that of Denise Lewis, did he actually list the criticisms. They were in essence that, 1: it was a 'case for section'; 2: labour went on too long and, 3: I had not delegated things properly.

111

The last case of the 4ft 10in teenager was not so alarming, *but there are serious features to it*.

In conclusion, two threads ran through the case against me; there were direct criticisms of my actions and decisions and, secondly, of their effect on the junior staff.

Apart from his opening remarks, it was a lacklustre performance. I had been told that Kennedy was a tough criminal barrister, but if he continued like this we ought to beat him hands down.

It was a strange experience to hear oneself criticised in public, but I knew that the first week would be the worst and I had to endure this before we could put the record straight.

We reviewed the day. The word incompetence had not been mentioned; the charges had not been listed. John thought Kennedy must find them an embarrassment. It could have been much worse. With some friends I went home to watch a TV programme, Panorama, about the case.

John had to read through his handwritten notes of Kennedy's opening speech and Brian went to sort out the affidavits that Hilary had been photocopying. Lawyers have a bad press, but I now understand that the court day is relatively short because of all the other work that has to be done.

Day 2. Tuesday, 4 February

The *Guardian* headline stretched right across page 2: 'Savage's "deficient care caused avoidable deaths"'; *The Times*: 'Obstetrician exposed mother and babies to danger, inquiry told'; the *Telegraph*: 'Babies' deaths "could have been avoided"'. But other papers changed the emphasis: 'Mothers' anger as Wendy faces "trial"', said the *Express* and 'Dr Wendy's big fight to win back her job', said the *Daily Mail*. I opened my encouraging post, took some blutack and thought I'd stick some of the postcards on the wall to cheer us up.

The morning started slowly; Mr Kennedy introduced Denise Lewis's letter complaining first about her notes being used without her permission and sent to all sorts of people, which she saw as a breach of the law of confidentiality, and secondly about the use of her case, as she had no complaints about her care, to prosecute me. Thirdly, she said that initials would not protect her confidentiality.

She ended by saying how angry she was that they had tried to use her to damage me. Mr Kennedy treated her complaint dismissively: *her notes are the property of the department, and we as the Health Authority have the custody and use of these . . . there is no question of this patient or that saying that they are not prepared to have their case examined because, after all, they do not have the knowledge that the profession have about whether this is right or wrong . . . desire for publicity has come from the other side . . . no wish to discuss in public.*

John Hendy made it clear that his instructing solicitor had spoken to her. She accepted that the publicity was now unavoidable but was still angry that her case was being used without her consent.

My up-to-date CV and an abbreviated one for Professor Grudzinskas were handed out. Kennedy took Grudzinskas through his 'evidence-in-chief' as it is called. He ran quickly through his CV and then the professor was asked to describe his philosophy about intervention: *Mr Kennedy, before I start, I would like to say at this point that only with extreme difficulty can I speak to this enquiry in public because, as a doctor, we are trained to consider matters concerning patients, and administrative matters relating to patients, as an aspect of serious confidentiality, and for that reason I prefer not to discuss any aspect of clinical matters, or the administrative related clinical matters, in public at all.*

I knew that unless the debate was public, even if I was exonerated, the destruction of my reputation would continue. Kennedy gave the chairman time to think about this request as he took Professor Grudzinskas through the 'philosophical' part of his evidence. Again he started off with an apologia, stressing that the London was not a high-tech unit, listing the area's social problems. Kennedy tried to put him at his ease and asked him about the 'old names' for Tower Hamlets. He didn't know them and I was allowed to tell the panel that Tower Hamlets included Stepney, Bow, Bethnal Green, Poplar and Spitalfields. Professor Grudzinskas stressed how counselling was used and parents' wishes always taken into account and how he had been associated with the equivalent to the National Childbirth Trust in Australia. I thought back to Mr Beaumont's words the previous day that 'only Mrs Savage is on trial' but the first hour of Gedis's testimony was devoted entirely to an attempt to defend and justify himself – eloquent evidence of the success of the press campaign. He then introduced the 1985 obstetric figures for intervention rates and perinatal mortality. The enquiry was supposed to be about my competence: would the chairman not intervene?

The outlining of the staffing, beds, duties and so on of the department took over an hour. Finally Kennedy moved on to the cases: *I suspect this is where you would like to discuss the sort of patients other than publicly?* It was a tense moment as the chairman turned to John Hendy: *The decision has been made that it should be conducted in public . . . My learned friend did open these matters in public.*

The members of the panel put their heads together as we watched anxiously. Finally the chairman straightened up: *We feel this evidence should be in public . . . I understand the professor's feelings, but he has done his duty.* As Mr Kennedy took Gedis through how the cases *came to his attention*, I made notes for John Hendy of where there were discrepancies between my recollection of the letters we had. We reached Susan Payne. Professor Howie brought up the question of whether or not it was a footling or a complete breech. I saw the chairman look puzzled. I whispered to John, 'Shall I get the pelvis?' He nodded. When I gave it and the doll to him, he offered it to Mr Kennedy via the chairman. Mr Kennedy looked at it without enthusiasm; Mr Dibley carried it across to the professor who pushed it away. Mr Beaumont said he thought a visual impression might be useful. Mr Kennedy: *Right. Can you put the baby into a complete breech?* The professor looked miserably at the pelvis. *Well, chairman, I have failed to put a baby into a complete breech using a doll on many occasions when I have tried before, and I have no reason to think that I can succeed now . . .* I watched him in amazement for it is something that most obstetricians teaching students do frequently; it really is quite easy to bend the soft doll's legs into any position you want to. Finally he put the doll into the position which fitted my drawing in the notes. Professor Howie: *That is what I would have said that a complete breech was.* Gedis: *Well, I regret, chairman, to disagree with Professor Howie . . . this doll may not accurately be representing what Professor Howie is trying to convey to us.* Then as he talks on he realises that he is describing a complete breech: *I would be guided by his view here.*

On and on it went. I could feel the women behind me watching these two professors having such difficulties in understanding each other. Mr Harvey could stand it no longer; he turned to the chairman and explained the differences between different kinds of breeches, concluding, . . . *I would accept this as a complete breech.* Peter

Howie was not to be deflected: *Is it possible that the X-rays may give us some help?* Mr Kennedy produced copies, the originals having been lost. Mr Harvey commented on the poor quality of the film: *It looks like a snowstorm.* Mr Beaumont: *So you both accept that it is a complete breech?* They did. Then Gedis said, *I shall be guided by the opinion of the enquiry. That is not a useful X-ray.* I wondered what had happened to the original after our copies had been made.

So the panel were doing our work for us, showing that the criticisms were not completely accurate. Laboriously, Gedis explained his criticisms of my care: the second stage was too long and I should not have used syntocinon. Then Mr Harvey asked if he would absolutely rule out the use of syntocinon in this woman. Gedis responded: *It is possible to consider a place for syntocinon usage in women in circumstances similar to this, but I do not think that in this instance, this instance was such an occasion when I would consider the use of syntocinon.* Kennedy tried again and Gedis launched into a lengthy explanation of how he would have used syntocinon in this woman only if she had been transferred to the theatre. I looked at him in amazement – the theatre, that cold clinical environment totally unsuitable for birth. Mr Harvey was looking at Professor Howie over Mr Beaumont's head.

Mr Kennedy did his best to repair the damage and after a few more questions about the timing of syntocinon which, after all, did not seem to be completely ruled out, he turned almost with relief to question Gedis about Linda Ganderson. Slowly and painfully we went through the notes. In short the staff didn't act when I was on holiday because they were confused.

On to AU, better photocopies of some pages were provided and handed around. The word counselling was used a lot when what Gedis meant was advice. At one point the chairman asked what was the difference between a trial of labour and a trial of scar. Mr Kennedy helped him out: *Your concern is whether it is going to get unzipped along the old scar line.* Again I felt conscious of the women behind me – so mechanical it sounded, not like one's uterus, the place where a child is nourished and grows. Gedis committed himself firmly about the cause of death: *It is extremely difficult to entertain any other possible cause here than some degree of trauma associated with the birth process.*

Denise Lewis came next, and after about an hour Professor Howie pointed out that one of the charges was 'factually incorrect':

the length of labour was given as fifteen hours. Mr Kennedy tried to work out how the mistake had occurred, that it should read eleven hours – as the criticism was about the length of labour. Professor Howie asked if it should still stand. Kennedy said he would have to consult his experts. It was never changed.

On to Ms X; again Professor Howie intervened to confirm that Gedis thought the trial of labour should have ended at 22.30 hours. *In my view yes.* Peter Howie, his fingertips together, leaned forward: *Could I put it to you that at that point the membranes were still intact, there was no caput succedaneum reported, and the registrar . . . thought that only two-fifths of the head was palpable. Now do you think on the basis of that you would be absolutely able to predict inability to deliver vaginally in safety?*

Gedis replied to the effect that he would not have got into that position in the first place. Mr Harvey then asked about X-ray pelvimetry and Gedis answered that, *In this respect, like many of the other views I share with Dr Savage, I would not have done an X-ray pelvimetry.* This differed from one of Gordon Bourne's criticisms.

I noted the way Gedis referred to me as *Doctor*, for in England as a whole obstetricians are considered as surgeons and called Mister rather than Doctor. Somehow there is a subtle downgrading of women obstetricians by referring to them like this rather than as Mrs, Miss or Ms. He had always called me Mrs Savage or Wendy before – why the Doctor all of a sudden? Mr Kennedy sat down. John Hendy rose, *Thank you*, he said, looking at Kennedy.

A short break was taken and we resumed at about 4 p.m. John Hendy stood up again. Mildly he asked whether these cases could be considered *unique, or is the sort of criticism raised in these cases, the sort of criticisms that might be raised on other obstetricians, in other circumstances, on other cases?* Gedis replied: *Chairman, is Mr Hendy actually referring to the collection of the cases – that is, the circumstances enclosed in the five particular cases?* John tried again: *The sort of criticisms which are raised in these five cases, are they criticisms which you think could be found on other cases dealt with by other obstetricians?* Gedis answered, *It is possible.*

John Hendy again: *Are they similar to criticisms which you feel that you could level at yourself looking back over your years as an obstetrician?* Gedis frowned, *If I can just consider that for a moment or two, chairman?* John replied, *Of course.* There was a long pause – everyone held their breath – *In specific detail, in specific clinical detail, it is possible in relation to at least one of the patient's cases that we are discussing here.* John paused to let this admission sink in and changed tack: *The way that these cases grew into the enquiry . . . is that you referred – yes, I think it was you – the case of AU to the District Medical Officer. Is that right?* Gedis reached for his glass: *I don't recall that to be the case.* John then asked, *That case, the case of AU, was referred to the DMO, and you were asked to express a view on it? Is that right?* Gedis pulled a file towards himself and began to leaf through the letters: *I was asked to express a view – I am referring to my notes here in order to be absolutely precise in my answers.* He turned the pages over, back and forth. I reflected that I had not seen him at close quarters since the previous summer. He looked uneasy; his hair had receded quite a bit. After what seemed an age he said he didn't have the correspondence in the file; he gave the impression that the District Medical Officer had asked him for reports but John made it clear that Gedis had volunteered some of them. Gedis said, *I believe that the DMO passed the reports . . . to the Regional Obstetric Assessor who I learned later was Gordon Bourne.* My sympathy evaporated: Gedis had been lecturer at Bart's, worked for Gordon Bourne, presumably read the Confidential Enquiries into Maternal Mortality which lists the Regional Assessors – Gordon Bourne had been one since 1974.

Soon after John asked, in the same even tone *When did you form the view that Mrs Savage was dangerous and incompetent?* A hush fell on the room. *I do not think, chairman, that I have ever expressed that view.* I heard an intake of breath behind me. *Does it follow it is not your view?* Gedis said how difficult he found it to speak publicly about *clinical matters, and the behaviour of my colleagues.* The chairman ruled firmly that the enquiry was a public enquiry and that I wanted it so and that John was putting questions on my behalf. Gedis replied: *Thank you. That is very helpful. It is difficult for me to answer the question directly in that it is so difficult to comment on who is dangerous and who is . . . I am not sure of the other word, Mr Hendy?* A gasp of incredulity ran round the upper benches, echoed by Mr Beaumont's *'incompetent' is the other word.* Gedis continued: *On who is dangerous and who is incompetent and when it occurs and how often it occurs and for how long it occurs at any particular time. It was my view that Dr Savage was an extremely hardworking individual with many, many, many commitments, and in the course of our discussions I urged her to consider a review of her many commitments so that she could give her important duties – in particular her heavy clinical duties – the attention they deserved. I sought the support of my other colleagues of the Medical College in the hospital in this respect.* I felt a sudden wave of anger, but it soon subsided; it was as if it was Gedis who was on trial today. And his reputation was not being enhanced.

Another long pause, then John said, *I'm sorry. That was your answer to the question, was it?*

Mr Kennedy produced the Particulars of Case which had been sent away for photocopying. *You were consulted over the formulation of those charges?* John asked. In a firmer voice Gedis replied, *That is correct.* Quietly and reasonably John asked him, *Does it follow that you are in general agreement with those charges?* Gedis agreed. The afternoon was over.

John Hendy had put the case clearly: it was about incompetence. We had a set of charges and the professor had been responsible for setting the case into motion. He handed the panel members the bundle of affidavits; they would have time to read them before the professor took his place on the witness stand the next day.

Day 3. Wednesday, 5 February

The *Guardian* headline read, 'Breach of confidence claim rejected' and a smaller 'Savage inquiry considers disputed evidence about "too long" labour'; *The Times*: 'Professor shared dilemma' and an editorial entitled 'Educating Patients' considered that an 'all-important cause had been served. It is the cause of professional demystification . . . doctors disagree even about fundamentals . . . at Mrs Savage's expense, their assent might in future be better informed.' I was glad that *The Times* thought it was important – but not quite sure how I felt at being the person on whom all this hinged.

John Hendy started this third day by going through the professor's CV, bringing out his relative lack of clinical work and his twelve years' experience against my twenty-five. I had realised that John would cross-examine their witnesses, but it was not until he began to ask Gedis about Professor Taylor's evidence that I understood that it was not all going to be their case against me in the first ten days. When I thought about it, it was obvious that the witness would have to be given a chance to reply to allegations that were going to be made – another part of the rules of evidence that I learnt as we went along.

John read from the affidavit '. . . *I can remember that on one occasion at the time of his appointment, he told me his first task was to change his senior lecturer. I know that he has expressed similar sentiments to other people.' That must be a matter of hearsay, but is it right you have expressed that view to other people?* Gedis described discussions about the Academic Unit and my role and the Medical College. John asked politely, *What is the short answer to the question, Professor Grudzinskas? Were you at the time of your appointment expressing the view that you wanted to get rid of Mrs Savage?* Gedis looked down at the floor: *Absolutely not* – but his voice dropped and the chairman had to ask him to repeat what he had said. This allegation was not new – it was in Professor Taylor's affidavit that we had used for the High Court proceedings some six months earlier. I was surprised that Gedis has not gone to greater lengths to refute it. If true, it would mean that all his evidence on the medical side would be open to attack as being influenced by personal bias, yet we had not received a sworn affidavit actually denying this on oath.

John then turned to the evidence of Peter Dunn, and read out part of his statement, made after he had read my colleagues' statements but before he had read the affidavits which made up the High Court case: . . . *'In a busy hospital misjudgements, failures in communication and frank mistakes are bound to occur to the best of doctors. It is usual to show understanding and sympathy when such events occur to a colleague, yet I find no trace of such support in any of the statements of Dr Savage's colleagues, which are not only highly critical, but tend to over-emphasise the adverse aspects, with at times the aid of hindsight. In no case is Dr Savage given the benefit of the doubt. In no case is the possibility that on occasion she might have been poorly served by her junior staff ever mentioned.' You can appreciate I do not want to ask you about this word for word but would you generally agree with the tone of that?*

Gedis replied, *No, I would not, but I would actually like to consider the precise wording of that letter, but the general theme I think is incorrect. I wouldn't agree.* A firm answer and John continued reading: *'I can say without hesitation that if the worst five of my own cases over the period of a year were put under a microscope, it would be possible to create a dossier similar to that of Mrs Savage. I believe the same could be done of every consultant obstetrician that I have ever worked with.'* Neonatal paediatricians probably know much more about obstetricians' practice than do fellow obstetricians, as they get the results of their work. I had been very encouraged when I had first seen this. The professor asked to have the paragraph read more slowly, then replied, *I think it is possible, chairman, to select the five worst cases of anybody, of any consultant in any discipline, and discuss the matter in some detail as can occur . . . could Mr Hendy read to me the latter part of the statement, because it is here some confusion arises in my mind.* John read the passage through again and Gedis responded, *I would not agree with this particular statement when we come to the word 'similar', because it is the dissimilarity in the clinical events that we are considering here, and which caused so much concern for these matters to come to the attention of the District Health Authority.*

Yet in June 1985 John Dennis, who was to be one of their expert witnesses, had expressed the view that it was the 'congruence' of these cases which led him to support my continued suspension – whereas here was Gedis saying it was their differences! John went on to deal with shared antenatal care, focusing on the 'agreed guidelines' which Gedis had mentioned the day before. This had been news to me as I thought we all had our own individual plans. Gedis produced a document; there was a pause while we looked at it. A murmur of astonishment ran around the room. He had produced a paper which dealt with home deliveries, a completely different subject! The chairman intervened, unusually revealing some impatience, and Gedis admitted that there were no written guidelines. Before going on to the issue of clinical autonomy, Gedis asked to be excused. I was quite glad of these breaks because of my period.

Professor, can I ask you whether you would agree with the proposition that Mrs Savage, like any other consultant, is not accountable either to you or to the Health Authority for the quality of her clinical judgement so long as she acts within the broad limits of acceptable medical practice? This was the cornerstone of our legal case and a fundamental principle of the NHS. Gedis, however, did not agree. *You disagree with that? In what respect do you disagree?*

In respect that her clinical practice may have implications on the academic responsibilities that the unit must discharge. Gedis expanded on this point that clinical autonomy is different in a teaching hospital. This will hardly go down well with those consultants, I thought. He continued, *In a teaching hospital it is necessary, I believe, for clinical autonomy to be considered in a different way from a non-teaching hospital.*

What does that mean? John Hendy asked. And Gedis replied, *Excuse me, Mr Chairman, what was the question?*

John rephrased Gedis's words and Gedis then agreed that, *if one holds an academic unit position, then the clinical autonomy may have to be modified.* I thought that this was an issue that senior lecturers throughout the country might unite on, and certainly explained his behaviour towards me. But after several more lengthy replies Gedis conceded that he meant I should explain my actions fully, and in answer to the question. John then asked, *What you are not suggesting is that any of the decisions that she makes should be modified because it is a teaching hospital?* Gedis replied, *No, I am not.* But maybe he was confused by the negatives!

Before he started on the cases John passed around my annual and study leave dates in 1984, and about 11.15 a.m. he began with Denise Lewis. We had gone through her case first because of the different clinical points and the 16 charges, although chronologically she was fourth on the list. It was a very shrewd legal move because it exposed the weakness of the case against me very clearly. John asked how my management of her anaemia demonstrated incompetence. Gedis said it didn't, then it did. The chairman tried to get him to give a straight answer. Inadequacies; then overseeing the management; I was responsible for what went on in the district; I should not have shared care with the GP. Mr Kennedy tried to help him out. Professor Howie intervened. With ruthless logic, John Hendy showed that the Charges 1 to 3 referring to shared antenatal care with the GP and investigation and treatment of the anaemia were nonsense: . . . *the first charge we can really strike out as far as you are concerned. That is not a demonstration of incompetence on her part.* John had already got Gedis to accept that shared care with the GP was a reasonable decision. I thought at last we would have the answer, yes. But instead: *In certain circumstances, no.*

Mr Beaumont: *Well, we are asking about these circumstances.* Gedis would not have chosen to share care. *I understand that but happily for you, your competence is not on trial – it is Mrs Savage's,* replied John. *You concede that she is not incompetent in prescribing this patient for shared care. It must follow . . . that Charge 1 against her can be struck out as far as your evidence is concerned from this charge sheet. No, I'm afraid not, sir,* Gedis responded. The initial decision to share care was not wrong, it should have been revised when seen by the registrar. Was I incompetent for leaving the decision to him? *No. So . . . where is the incompetence in relation to Mrs Savage in relation to shared care?*

Sir, may I come back to the question of consultant responsibility here, in that in my mind the deficiency here is that there does not seem to have been an adequate consideration of the suitability of this lady continuing her care in a shared care system which would provide for her medical needs satisfactorily.

John decided to move on to pre-eclampsia. He demolished the fourth charge, alleging that Denise had severe pre-eclampsia in June. Then to the 5 July note: again Gedis's criticisms were difficult to pin down. It was a relief to us all when 4.30 came.

We discussed the day. We had only gone through four of the fifty-nine charges with one of their witnesses. John said that it would be quicker after today but I was worried about the slowness of Gedis's evidence.

I drove to the hospital, collected my mail and, seeing Sid Watkins's car in the consultant's car park, went to see him to ask if there was any way that the district's case could be speeded up. As I walked through the door into the Alexandra Wing, Gedis passed me, walking hurriedly and looking anxious. Sid's door was open; I told him my fears about the slow progress and he said they were shared by the professor. That was a relief to me. When I had been in Mr Dibley's office in December he had told me that they had set aside four weeks because if we weren't finished in two it might take months to reconvene the panel and lawyers. I could not face the thought of another six months' suspension from my work.

Day 4. Thursday, 6 February

'Hospital chief "wanted Savage out as lecturer" – replacing accused consultant was seen as first task' was the *Guardian* headline with a picture of Professor Grudzinskas who 'helped to draw up charges'. *The Times*, 'Savage plot is denied'.

As I drove into the car park at Addison House, it was still grey and cold. I saw Gedis arriving in a taxi with the thick-set man who, although he looked like a heavyweight boxer, I had discovered was the MPS solicitor. Gedis looked less worried than the night before.

I decided to show how intervention in birth at the London Hospital was rising, and the number of deliveries by consultant, just to get the record straight. And now that the obstetric figures for 1985 had been introduced, it seemed likely that we could also introduce figures. I took the London Hospital annual obstetric reports and piled them up on our desk and drew up some graphs whilst listening to the cross-examination.

We started at 9.30 a.m. and John Hendy took Gedis rapidly through the rest of Denise Lewis's notes – the birth plan interpreted as a set of inflexible instructions, but not well enough defined, according to Gedis, who would not accept that I could have expected the senior registrar to use his discretion. John asked, *You are suggesting, are you, that she should have explicitly set out all the options, and the factors to be taken into account in deciding for and against each or something?* The professor replied, *That would have been one way of dealing with the situation, yes.* But he did not accept that this was – *a counsel of perfection in a busy hospital?* The professor did not.

Susan Payne was discussed next. John took him methodically through the charges. Gedis said that the reason that syntocinon should not be given with a breech was the risk of feto-pelvic disproportion. But he was reluctant to accept that this risk was negligible although, finally, he agreed that in a woman with a large pelvis like this, syntocinon was not ruled out – thus getting Charge 2 out of the way.

We moved on to Linda Ganderson. Gedis betrayed his unfamiliarity with the Dundee chart (an ultra-sound chart to show fetal growth) which has been in use in our district since 1982. He questioned its validity. The point of this chart was that it showed that the GP's note on 12 March 'Wrong dates likely' was a perfectly reasonable conclusion and that there was no need in the circumstances to admit Linda to hospital, *at thirty weeks . . . or at the very latest 12.3.84*, as had been one of the charges against me.

Gedis admitted that the chances of the baby surviving would have been high if delivered on 18 April and that he knew that I was on holiday then.

In the case of AU, John attempted to summarise the eight charges running to over two A4 pages: *the essence of what is said against Mrs Savage here is that there should have been no trial of labour? . . .* Gedis agreed: *I think that tends to summarise what is in the particulars of the case.* It was mid-afternoon; the close air in the dimly lit chamber made us all feel tired. I noticed Mr Kennedy looking at Gedis with a detached, almost quizzical air. We turned to the compendium and John returned to his original question about trial of labour. Again, by a series of logical questions, John showed that Gedis did not support all the charges. We went through the notes line by line, decision by decision. Professor Howie intervened to clarify whether Charge 2(i) should stand after Gedis had said that AU need *not* have had an elective Caesarean.

At about 3.45 p.m. we reached Ms X. Over and over again John tried to get the professor to define in what way the trial of labour carried out was *not* a trial of labour, as stated in Charge 1. The chairman tried to help. As to the delivery, Mr Beaumont asked: *Was it wrong for Mrs Savage to leave it to Dr Robinson?* Without hesitation Gedis replied, *I believe so, yes*. But four questions later he agreed that it would depend on what information I had had from the registrar.

The afternoon was finally over.

Day 5. Friday, 7 February
Nothing in the *Guardian*. 'Experts clash on birth', said *The Times*.

That morning John introduced the graphs which I had drawn, the deliveries by consultant and the perinatal figures I had submitted to the DHA the previous June. Gedis looked puzzled and said he'd never seen the latter before, although on questioning he agreed that he'd seen the report in *The Times*. (Nicholas Timmins had quoted the figures I'd given to the DHA, saying that 'her perinatal death rate in the 16 months to April 1985 was 11.3 against an average of 13.7 for the other four consultants at the same hospital'.

John tied up a few ends; on sessions, Gedis was uncertain; Was the community antenatal care scheme at risk? Mr Kennedy attempted to repair the damage – but Gedis stated that there was no time for consultants to go into the community. We would need another consultant. Mr Beaumont asked if there was anyone doing my work. Gedis replied that there was a locum but she was not doing all the work. He left the witness table after three days and half a morning.

Next came Mr and Mrs U. I was saddened to see them – I felt and still feel both anger and regret that I have been unable to help them with their understandable grief. After lunch the two senior house officers involved with Denise Lewis, one also with Mrs U, gave evidence. I expected the professor or Mr Conlin to ask if they could give their evidence in camera – and I would not have objected at all – but they did not. It was a relief, they answered 'yes', 'no' and 'I don't know'. If they couldn't remember they said so and their evidence confirmed mine on several points. And neither of them said they were confused by my management.

We finished at 4 p.m. The first week was over and now things ought to move faster. We weighed it up: the chairman had not drawn the terms of reference narrowly; we had introduced the affidavits; John had shown up the paucity of their case. The professor had been unimpressive; we had introduced the perinatal figures. And the press coverage, apart from the first day, had been better than expected. So far so good. There was some anxiety about time; Kennedy had said they needed ten working days for their witnesses, but he had been so slow – and so had the professor. Would we have time for all of ours?

The following day the *Guardian* headline was: 'Consultants end pioneering scheme for community care of pregnant women'. *The Times* and the *Telegraph* had picked up the perinatal mortality figures: ' "Fewer babies" were lost by obstetrician' and 'Obstetrician had the best success rate', the former I accepted, the latter was not scientifically accurate without more data analysis! It was not until I really knew the details of what was being reported that I understood the power of the subtitle writers and how infuriating it must be for the responsible journalist to have his carefully worded report appearing under a 'sensational' headline.

I started to reply to the letters and cards that had come during the week. Many people had sent cheques as well. It was good to feel supported.

· CHAPTER 11 ·

Expert Witnesses for the Prosecution

It is the customary fate of new truths to begin as heresies and to end as superstitions.

T. H. Huxley, *Collected Essays*

Mr Nysenbaum, the lecturer, was a very confident witness, but there was considerable discrepancy between his recollections of when we met with the Us at 8.30 in the morning in the labour ward and mine. Fortunately for me the evidence of the SHO and Dr Fay differed from his memories. At the end of his evidence on the Monday afternoon, Mr Kennedy asked him about another woman – nothing to do with the five named in the terms of reference. John Hendy objected; the public were sent out and although John argued strongly against this, Mr Kennedy said that this was evidence to back up the general charges that my management was confusing to the junior staff. His plea was accepted, and everyone trooped back in. There had been some mention of this case before lunch and over the meal I had told John and Brian all about her: I recalled her name, her considerable social problems, her severe pre-eclampsia, a violent partner, possible drug addiction, threats to 'thump' the staff, and how angry I had been when Tony Nysenbaum had refused to carry out my instructions. I had spoken to him late the following evening and kept a record of the conversation in August 1984. He had described my management as 'dangerous', but had withdrawn the remark after I had said I found it offensive. After this conversation I had had no further difficulties with Tony.

Kennedy took him through this case and all Tony could remember about the woman was that he had refused to give her intravenous prostaglandin when I had asked for this to be done. In cross-examination he said that he had done this *eyeball to eyeball* whereas I remembered him ringing me in the antenatal clinic.

To me this exemplified the difference in approach which I felt divided me from some of my colleagues: Tony had no memory of the woman or the obstetric problems in her case – just the use of the drug prostaglandin. I remembered him saying that she ought to have a Caesarean, not that the dispute was about the drug. I remembered vividly the labour, the social problems and how I had delivered her. At the end of the day, I drove to Mile End, went to the records department and got the case notes. I then rang Jean Richards, and said they had raised a sixth case and I wanted to take the notes in to the enquiry the next day. She sounded shocked but agreed. Then I went and sat down in the labour ward and went through the delivery book, counting the number of patients of mine that Tony Nysenbaum had looked after before and after this episode. This confirmed my recollection that there were no other 'problem cases'. I got home at 10.30 p.m. It had been nice to see the midwives, and one of my patients had delivered whilst I was there, though I didn't go into her room.

The other junior staff did not give any evidence to support Mr Kennedy's case that I had confused them, and some of their evidence was very helpful for my defence. For example, Toby Fay, the registrar who had spoken with the Us at 4 and 5.30 in the morning of 26 April 1984, confirmed that he had put the options of Caesarean section or trial of labour to them – the pros and the cons – that Mrs U was not in labour at that time, that I liked to be kept informed, and that I usually knew about my patients, although he thought I had unconventional views.

John Dennis, Professor of Obstetrics and Gynaecology, University of Southampton: The first of their expert witnesses was John Dennis, who like so many distinguished obstetricians had trained in Aberdeen in the days of Sir Dugald Baird. He is a short man, and was very relaxed in the witness chair, a complete contrast to Gedis. He gave his evidence in a conversational tone, talking to the panel members as if in a hospital rather than a courtroom. But under cross-examination he was not impressive. His emphasis on protocols; no problems in his unit once the oldest consultant had retired; his labelling of women at booking on the basis of risk factors betrayed a rigidity of approach which at times I found oppressive. Professor Howie asked him: *Do you think that enforced uniformity could be a barrier to progress?* His answer: *If it is never analysed or reviewed, of course,* suggested to me that innovation would be unlikely to happen in his unit.

Taking up a point from his second letter to Dr Richards on my workload John asked him, *Would it be right to take from your evidence that she is a lady who is, as an obstetrician, incompetent?* He replied, *It is impossible to answer that, because for that I would really have to know much more about the rest of her work. So I cannot – I'm not saying yes and I'm not saying no. I do not know.* I looked at him with new eyes. This was the man who wrote those damning words 'bizarre and incompetent', 'consistent aberration of clinical judgement', but when asked a direct question he wouldn't commit himself.

That is a very cautious answer, professor. He smiled at John. *It has to be.* He admitted that unless you worked closely with someone it was hard to judge, he had a lot of sympathy with many of the things I stood for, he wondered how incompetence was defined. Everybody laughed.

John tried a different tack: *Mrs Savage was suspended, or part of the basis for the suspension was that she was dangerous. It would have been dangerous if she had continued in office as it were. Are you able to express a view? Would you agree that she was dangerous on the basis of the notes that you have seen?* There was a pause. *Dangerous is a strong word.* He circled round the point. *I am avoiding the word dangerous.*

Throughout the cross-examination, I passed John notes covering various points under discussion. John glanced down at one of the notes and remarked: *We know that dysfunctional labour is often a manifestation of disproportion, is that right, professor? Is dysfunctional labour a manifestation of disproportion in a multiparous woman?* Dennis frowned: *Not usually, unless, of course –* he paused – *I cannot remember now how far she progressed in her first labour . . .* John asked astutely, *It got to 4½ cm . . . how would that affect it?* Dennis replied, *The uterus is then more likely to function like a primigravid uterus than a multiparous one.* He leaned back in his chair. John pressed him further, *Is that a view based on research?* Dennis twisted a little in the chair: *No, it's not. Just experience.*

There was quite a lot of laughter during the two days of his evidence, but there was one point where every woman in the room shuddered with distaste. Ian Kennedy was asking him about Susan Payne's long second stage. He responded, *I myself have extended the second stage in a breech delivery on a few occasions, but I was sitting beside the patient.* Kennedy smiled down at him: *Literally?* Dennis turned towards him and said, *Well, at the bottom end.* They both sniggered. Again it emphasised the gulf between the two sides of the room.

He thought the majority of British obstetricians would not allow a trial of labour with a scar in the uterus if the inlet of the pelvis was under 10 cm but conceded that at thirty-four weeks he might if the head was well down in the pelvis. He thought that a baby of 2.6 kg was the largest that would safely go through an inlet of 9.75. (There is published evidence that a breech baby of this weight can pass safely and if it is head first, it can weigh as much as 2.9 kg.) He retracted his earlier allegation about 'imminent eclampsia' by redefining it: *It does not mean to say that eclampsia is going to happen in a minute or two.* (Doesn't it? I teach the students that it requires urgent action because fits may occur at any time.)

He accepted that the pre-eclampsia was not severe in June, that the criticism of the management of the anaemia not being treated energetically was not a severe censure. But despite this, when asked by John Hendy if his agreement to Charges 6, 7 and 9 in Denise Lewis *does do justice to your position?* he changed ground again. *The problem about this investigation is that things have to be put in black and white, and given the limits of this process I agree with 6, 7 and 9.* I looked at him in amazement. Didn't he realise that this 'process' had prevented me from working for forty-one weeks and could destroy my professional reputation and career for ever?

Lastly John reached the case of AU: *Your criticism there is that in spite of adverse signs, Mrs Savage decided to continue with a trial of labour.* Dennis refined his criticism: *The possibility of vaginal delivery, yes.* John: *That is really the only clinical decision that you challenge on Mrs Savage's part.* Dennis: *Well, as I said in my original summary, all the other cases apart from AU could have occurred. I could have seen those in the practice of many other consultants.*

So it seemed to me that unless the other consultants were incompetent or all practising 'outside the limits of acceptable medical practice' he had destroyed the Health Authority's case, as earlier he had said that one case could not be used to prove incompetence. John: *Of the other cases you say it is the congruence of these cases which troubles you, but now having examined each one of them, the panel may find it difficult to understand how the congruence of these cases reveals anything about the competence of Mrs Savage at all.* Professor Dennis shifted his position in his chair. He looked uneasy for the first time. *We are all human and we can all make mistakes. It is the frequency with which we make errors which reveals our overall competence.*

Professor, that goes without saying. That is understandable, but where the errors, so-called, amount merely to what is demonstrated in those four other cases, and where the errors, so-called, are so different in nature, they really do not reveal anything about Mrs Savage's competence at all, do they? Professor Dennis turned towards the dais: *Well, that is for the panel to decide.* Very quietly John said to him, *It is also for you to express an opinion about.* Professor Dennis looked at him: *Well, I think if I put it another way, had there only been the four cases, I think the conclusions I would have reached would have been different. Would that satisfy your question?*

I am a hard man to satisfy, professor. Your emphasis on the congruence might be understood if all the so-called errors in these cases were of the same nature, if they were all failures to intervene with a Caesarean section, or if they were a consistent pattern of lack of instruction to general practitioners for antenatal care. But those four cases other than AU all demonstrate different things, do they not? John Dennis looked down again: *Well, yes. I think that two of them have a hint of reluctance to do a Caesarean section apart from AU as well. Three altogether have that.* He leaned back again, crossing his legs. *But apart from that there is not a lot of similarity between them? No that is right.*

John read out the passage in Professor Dennis's second letter about reducing my workload, having established that perhaps the whole workload of the district might be looked at to see if some people were doing too little rather than it being me at fault for doing too much. And then he said, *Can we take it from what you say that the very last thing you would recommend is that this lady should be dismissed on grounds of incompetence?*

If all the evidence of incompetence is encompassed by what has been discussed here, I would be sad to see that. John pressed him a bit harder: *More than sad, it would not be right, would it?* Dennis shifted in the chair again: *I think I will leave the panel to judge that.* I wondered if he had ever been responsible for assessing a consultant's competence before – he looked glad that he was not the one to make a decision – but it was his report in June that had enabled the Chairman of the DHA to maintain my suspension.

Gordon Bourne, Regional Assessor for Maternal Mortality: Gordon arrived on day 11, Monday 17 February. I had not seen him since just before I was suspended – we used to meet once a month at Bart's as part of the Joint Academic Unit along with Gedis and Tim Chard and the Bart's consultants. In my affidavit Brian had translated what I had said about his attitude to me into 'had displayed personal animosity towards me' and in the rush I had not corrected this. I felt I owed him an apology: I greeted him and said I was sorry – the statement was not quite accurate. He had always been perfectly polite. We chatted together amicably until Trevor Beedham sat down as the panel filed in.

Gordon Bourne took the stand just before lunch. In his well-cut suit, with the carnation in the button hole, and greying hair, although looking younger than his sixty-five years, he is a typical Harley Street obstetrician. Retired Senior Consultant at Bart's, he had also worked at the Royal Masonic Hospital. He answered the questions in a very soft voice, almost inaudible at times, with an occasional intonation of the vowels which reflected his North Country origins.

We stopped for lunch. By chance I was behind him in the queue: 'Not much fun.' 'No,' I replied, 'it's rather like a viva, isn't it?' 'Rather a long one,' he looked uneasy. I replied deliberately, 'Yes, Gedis looked pretty sick after three and a half days in the witness box.' Ahead of us, Gedis was collecting his plate, talking to one of the lawyers. He looked completely relaxed. I wondered what was going on inside his head. That afternoon Kennedy took Gordon Bourne through his evidence. He talked rapidly, fluently, his speech peppered with words like disaster, dangerous, dire consequences, life of baby at stake. His position at one end of the spectrum of obstetric opinion emerged more and more clearly: *No woman should ever be allowed to go into labour with a haemoglobin under 10 Gms'*. He dismissed the risks of antenatal X-rays even when pressed by Professor Howie, although he retracted his criticism that there had not been satisfactory antenatal assessment of the pelvis when Howie pushed him harder. *I accept absolutely that a clinical pelvimetry done by a consultant on this patient is perfectly acceptable.* The charge about fetal distress he also retracted after Professor Howie had intervened. With AU he would have strongly warned the husband of the dangers: *rupturing her uterus . . . the life of his child is indeed at very, very grave risk*. He ended by saying in that characteristically mild voice (it sounds so reasonable that one almost doesn't hear the strong words), the dire threats, the ominous fears, the undercurrent of anxiety about normal pregnancy: *the messages tend to be different, don't they* – he is discussing my style of management, so he doesn't agree with John Dennis. *There is somewhere a lack of responding to warning signals and lack of reaction to situations that may become dangerous and in some instances do . . . if there is a theme here it is a lack of reaction to conditions which might have been – or in some circumstances should have been, responded to.*

Brian had decided, with John Hendy's agreement, to cross-examine Mr Bourne the next day, a move that Mr Kennedy obviously regarded with suspicion. John Hendy was not a QC and now a mere solicitor conducting a cross-examination – it was like asking the SHO to take a consultant to task!

Brian, assisted by Peter Howie, who intervened more than he had done before, exposed the rigid, authoritarian view of obstetric practice that Mr Bourne represented: the treatment of Denise Lewis's anaemia was outside accepted limits; women with pre-eclampsia should stay in hospital; it was difficult to draw the line between severe pre-eclampsia and eclampsia. For a woman to go past thirty-eight weeks with a haemoglobin less than 9 Gms was dangerous. Acceptable practice was what was in student textbooks and standard practice in teaching hospitals – although he did modify this after Mr Beaumont pressed him near the end of the day. No wonder the professor and the lecturer who had both worked for him were so 'anxious' and saw as 'dangerous' plans of management which deviated from the narrow pathway they had been taken along by Mr Bourne.

Brian put it to him that he was wrong about his view about the spectrum of practice in the profession at large. *No, I'm not,* he said more firmly than anything else that day. But he could not accept that in Ms X Professor Dennis had said there was no case to answer. *Would it be impertinent of me to say that Professor Dennis is at fault?* There was a burst of laughter from behind me. Mr Kennedy looked annoyed. The professor, sitting staring into space, did not react.

At one point Bourne showed emotion, delivering a lecture about Linda's baby: *These are the babies that die,* he said in a choked voice (and without any good scientific evidence). *I'm sorry . . . I didn't mean to bang the table.* It was an impressive performance, but it left me cold. I remembered those who had told me about Gordon

Bourne's skill at politics, his charming manner towards me whenever we had met, in contrast to his role in my suspension, to which Brian now turned. He denied that he had anything to do with it despite Jean Richards' letter of 26 September 1984 asking him to look at the case reports to see 'whether there was a *prima facie* case for suspension', and the tone of his own affidavit in August 1985 (both Mr Kennedy and Mr Conlin objected to this line of questioning by Brian). Brian then tried to establish exactly how Mr Bourne had approached the task of assessing the cases – obviously a sensitive area. Mr Kennedy kept leaping to his feet like a jack-in-the-box and Mr Conlin, in contrast, quietly glided up when he intervened. Clearly here was a difference in the way the panel reacted: Peter Howie did not look convinced by many of Gordon Bourne's answers to his questions and could see that there was an important point here and wanted to pursue it. The chairman backed the lawyers on the other side. And Len Harvey leaned back, fingering his unlit pipe.

The day finished with Mr Bourne saying he had used the word 'mismanagement' advisedly, but, *putting life at risk or in jeopardy was one definition of incompetence.* He agreed with Mr Harvey that there had to be persistence of error and here the underlying philosophy was important. He accepted Professor Howie's point about acknowledgement of error needing to be taken into account. Mr Beaumont then asked, *So you can envisage circumstances in which competent practice could be something other than that which is set out in the standard textbooks and teaching practice?*

Yes, sir. Because that is really the only way we move. Had he realised that the answer he had given so firmly to Brian six hours before put him out on a limb? Mr Beaumont looked at him benignly: *That is the way medicine advances.* Mr Bourne smiled at him in return: *That is the only way we move forward.*

That completed their expert witnesses' evidence and we did not think that they had produced a very convincing case. But this is where Mr Kennedy would come into his own in trying to break me and then discredit our expert witnesses. He was not familiar with the notes and from his line of questioning it looked as if he had almost abandoned many of the original fifty-nine Charges and was busy constructing a new case.

On Friday evening the lawyers had decided to look into the possibility of extending the hours we worked and the next week it was agreed to do this; then, as the time still seemed insufficient, to sit for another week. Five weeks for five cases – it seemed incredible. But the legal process was extremely slow and tortuous – and Mr Kennedy's stubborn attempts to win his case extended this. At the end of the prosecution case I felt how ridiculous it was to continue. But part of me wanted to show clearly what the defence was and another part of me knew that once the system was set, it had to go through all the motions, however nonsensical they seemed.

· CHAPTER 12 ·

I Defend my Practice

It is not ultimately a matter of High Tech versus natural childbirth. The doctor does not necessarily always know best. A woman having a baby is doing what she was designed for and that equips her with a kind of knowing. Surely humility and respect on both sides is what is needed . . . The awareness of the paper-thin divide between life and death can be life-enhancing or can shake your confidence completely.

Mary Ellis, *British Medical Journal*, 25 January 1986

The case for the prosecution ended just after lunch on Wednesday 19 February – the last lunch I was to have with Brian and John until I had finished giving my evidence. It seemed to be an extraordinary rule that, during this time, when I needed them most, I discovered that I was not allowed to speak about the case to my legal advisers – but that is how the system works!

The Defence Case Opens

After lunch on day 13 of the enquiry, John Hendy rose to present our side of the case. I looked across to Mr Kennedy; he looked almost bored, leaning with his back towards the professor sitting in the second row, expressionless, almost as if he were detached from the proceedings. Kennedy now looked at the panel, and I supposed he was watching them for signs of reaction to John's opening speech. I thought about the differences between their two voices: Kennedy had that plummy, public-school, accented voice and used phrases like 'jolly good'. When his line of questioning had not produced the desired results he would say, 'Very well' in a curt tone. John Hendy, on the other hand, had a neutral accent with occasional words that reminded one of his West London background. He began his speech by presenting extracts from my comments to the chairman which had been drafted very lucidly by Brian the summer before. This set the scene. John defined incompetence very clearly, and then pointed out that imperfection was not uncommon in medical practice, however hard doctors tried. He then outlined what was left of the prosecution case: he dismissed Ms X – there was no case to answer, according to one of the two Health Authority experts, but what of the others? In the case of Susan Payne, was I incompetent because I decided to wait and see how the labour progressed in a woman with a large pelvis? As for Linda Ganderson, was I incompetent because I had not ordered a first-trimester scan and had delegated care to the GP? And regarding Denise Lewis, was I incompetent because I had not ordered prophylactic iron and folic acid, had I ignored the pre-eclampsia, and was it incompetent to induce with syntocinon? He said I would admit that I had not written this note perfectly, but was it incompetent to ask the senior registrar to 'sort it out', i.e. use his discretion?

In the case of AU they had to decide whether I was incompetent to ask Toby Fay to speak to the woman at 4.30 in the morning, to decide on a trial of labour at 8.30 and to continue it at 12.15 p.m. As for the allegation that *my conduct of the cases confused junior staff, there was not a shred of evidence to support that.* It was said that I failed to appreciate or understand the risks involved, but in fact I was an obstetrician who weighed up every risk; it was also said that I lacked insight because I referred to the good outcome in three of the cases, but this was absurd.

I Speak for Myself

Finally, it was my turn to speak. I was to give my account of the management of these cases after exactly forty-three weeks of suspension, and after two weeks of hearing other people's criticisms of the way the cases had been handled. I walked to the table and sat in the chair where I was to sit for the next week, facing the panel, with John Hendy and Brian Raymond on my left and Mr Kennedy and James Badenoch on my right. I couldn't see my supporters very well because of the subdued lighting, but I could feel their presence behind me. The press benches were almost as full as they had been on the first day.

John took me through my curriculum vitae, my philosophy and attitude to childbirth, my timetable at work, what I knew about the setting-up of the HM (61) 112 and the collection of the cases. I felt quite relaxed because of the work that we had done and the way that John had such a clear and thorough grasp of the case. As he asked the questions (which we had not rehearsed), I was very glad that I had changed to Brian Raymond; I felt that not only had I got good lawyers but that we understood each other. It was a bit like being interviewed on radio or television: when you feel on the same wavelength as the interviewer, the programme goes well.

The next morning the headlines differed. The *Guardian* had 'Savage spells out her case'; *The Times* 'Savage a victim of colleagues', the *Telegraph* 'Men frightened of birth pains' and the *Daily Mail* 'Natural birth doctor answers critics'. My age, which had been reported as lower and lower since I had been suspended and had reached forty-two, was now correctly given as fifty. All four of the papers had also quoted part of my answer to John's questions about my approach to obstetrics: . . . *I think that obstetrics spans the whole spectrum of attitudes from what I call the 'pessimistic approach', that no labour is normal except in retrospect – and I believe that Mr Bourne and Professor Dennis tend to that end of the spectrum – to the other end which I call the 'optimistic approach', which I think reflects my own personality, that everything is normal until something goes wrong. Pregnancy is not an illness. It is a very important part of a woman's life, a couple's life together, and it is of enormous psychosocial significance. I think that it is very important that the people who are assisting a woman during pregnancy allow her to feel in control of the situation and not feel taken over by the hospital, by the doctor, by the system, because if she does feel that way, she is far less able to be this autonomous new person who is a parent.*

John asked me how the two views differed in practice. I referred to John Dennis labelling women as high-risk, preventing them from feeling that they were healthy pregnant women (although obviously some women did need extra special care, but you had to be careful not to label almost all women as being 'high risk'). *What about the male/female approach you referred to just now?*

I think that men, who are not going to actually physically give birth, but are onlookers and bystanders, have the feeling that they have got to do something about the pain, about the way labour is progressing, whereas women, who know that they will probably go through this experience, even if they have not already been through it, understand that it is a very important part of how a woman functions in life, and that there are worse things in life than pain, and that to go through the process of pregnancy and labour and be in control of it is a very important part of a woman's self-esteem. Now, I did not learn that from my own experience of giving birth, I must say. I learned it from women that I

*looked after. And most notably from Peter Huntingford when I came to work
for him in 1976.*

Day 14. Thursday, 20 February. I Transgress the Rules of Evidence

We started at 10.15 a.m. Both Mr Kennedy and Mr Beaumont had
travelled in by train from the country and had been held up by the
wintry weather. It was when John had asked me about the Trevor
Beedham letter of 21 May 1984 that Mr Harvey asked me a
question which I found really upsetting. We had been discussing
the phone calls which had gone on behind the scenes, when he
suddenly said to me, in his quiet unemotional voice, *Did you find that
a little sad, that Dr Fay had not communicated with you?* I *had* found it very
sad, and I had been even more saddened as I had listened to his
evidence because I felt so terrible that the junior staff should have
been mixed up in all this struggle among their seniors. I answered
noncommittally, and then he asked me if I had had it out with Mr
Fay. I suddenly remembered, vividly, speaking to Toby on 22 May
after I had received Mr Beedham's letter.

I forgot I was sitting in this room, surrounded by lawyers, the
press, my judges and women, I just remembered the feelings and
the conversation, and I recounted it as I recalled it: *I said to him, 'I
do not think that this baby died because of her labour or because of her delivery
and I think this baby died because of a rare blood disorder.' He was obviously
upset about it, and feeling responsible about it, and I said to him, 'Look, I
knew I could trust you to put across the case of having a Caesar or having a
vaginal delivery because I knew that you wanted – you thought it was the
correct thing to do a Caesarean section so you were not going to be pushing the
vaginal delivery aspect.' And he said to me, 'But you know, I didn't want to do
any Caesar because I was tired.'* When I had finished there was a
moment's silence and then Mr Kennedy was on his feet. His
objection – which was only later explained to me – was that the
normal court rules of evidence require the defendant's case to be
put to the witnesses on the other side so that they can 'put their
case', and because I had never discussed this conversation with my
lawyers, and it was not part of our defence, I had transgressed the
rules. But I was unaware of this, so was completely confused by all
the fuss.

With all this talk of points and Mr Conlin also rising to his feet, I
saw that they were all taking this remark as being a criticism. But

that was not how it was meant. I wished I had never spoken, all my feelings about the disruption of the relationships with the junior staff and midwives, the way pressure had been put on them not to talk to me or go on marches, the suspicion in the department, the division of loyalties, the split between the GPs and the obstetricians in the district, the gynae ward shut – that terrific team of nurses disbanded. These thoughts flashed through my mind as I heard the lawyers discussing whether to recall Mr Fay. As they finished, I said to the chairman, *I'm sorry that Mr Harvey asked that question. I do not think that I have ever discussed that conversation with Brian Raymond or John Hendy. It was just . . .* I could not go on. I thought that I was going to cry – I fought the tears back; I couldn't cry here, it wasn't the right time or the right place. Mr Beaumont helped me out: *Sometimes things do come out that have not been anticipated.* I asked the press not to put that remark in, as I hadn't discussed it with Toby and Mr Beaumont reinforced my plea.

The rest of that day was taken up by my evidence about Susan Payne, Linda Ganderson and Denise Lewis. John Hendy took me through each case, but the obstetricians on the panel also asked me questions, so that it was much less like a trial and more like a viva or at times even a discussion between professionals.

That evening I went to collect my mail at Whitechapel, and met Toby Fay in the lift. I said I was sorry that he had had to come back, but I supposed that it would be wrong of me to explain the reasons, as we were in the middle of this legal battle. I wish now that I had explained things, because it might have limited the damage.

Day 15. Friday, 21 February. Emotions, Fatigue and Training

Guardian: 'Savage felt isolated from decisions'; *The Times*: '"I was isolated", Savage tells inquiry'. I read the *Guardian* article while waiting for the kettle to boil. It wasn't by Andy Veitch but by someone I had never met, and right at the end he had put in the quote, as had Nick Timmins in *The Times*, which I had hoped they would not.

Reading those articles was bad enough, but the atmosphere in the chamber was even worse. John Hendy asked Toby Fay about my statement: *Do you remember saying words to the effect that in your heart of hearts one of the reasons connected with you not doing a Caesar during the early hours of the morning was that you were tired?* Toby Fay replied: *That's not it* and John Hendy continued: *The only question that arises from that: was it, in fact, the case that, on the night before the delivery of the AU baby, you were tired?* Toby Fay: *I am always tired!* There was a burst of sympathetic laughter from those in the audience who included that morning some GPs who had done SHO jobs in our department, but Toby did not pick up the fellow feeling and said somewhat defensively, *Most of the junior registrars are.*

John Hendy: *Was that a reason for doing or not doing anything in particular in relation to that?* Toby Fay: *Absolutely not, and I think the implication is –* he paused and he sounded angry – *the implication of saying that I would not do something because I was tired is not right.* John Hendy: *And something you would resist?* Toby Fay: *And resent, I might add.*

Mr Conlin rose to his feet: *With your leave, with the greatest respect to my learned friend, Mr Hendy, I submit it is not putting properly what Mrs Savage said in the witness box yesterday.* Mr Kennedy stood up and said, *It is not, but the ground, I observe, is moving. What she said in the witness box yesterday was: 'He said, "I did not want to do another Caesar because I was tired."'* There was no question of shilly-shallying yesterday.

At that moment I could have shaken Mr Kennedy. The words were the same but the mood, the emotion behind them were quite different. My attempt to convey the emotional nuances of a conversation two years ago was twisted and thrown back at me. His tone said it all: I was lying, prevaricating, shifting my ground in order to hide the truth. We were not taking part in a dispassionate scientific enquiry – this was the Old Bailey style at its worst.

Although John tried hard to state clearly on my behalf that no criticism of Mr Fay was intended, I could see he felt criticised; he would not look at me. Later I tried to repair the damage when I came back to give my evidence-in-chief. John gave me the opportunity: *I think you had better tell us your best recollection of that conversation.* I started by speaking about the emotion experienced in a department when a baby dies. I then repeated the conversation I'd had with Toby when I remembered him saying that he did not really want to do a Caesarean because he was tired. I continued: *We both knew that often when you are woken up in the middle of the night, in your heart of hearts all you want to do is to turn over and go to sleep. But your professional*

*training overcomes that, and you get up and you do go in and you do the
Caesarean section or whatever. In no way did I think that Toby was reluctant
to do the Caesarean section. When you have conversations like this, they are not
really for public discussion. They are sensitive and about emotions, and they do
not take well to being dealt with in this kind of forum and being reported in
newspapers, which, after all, summarise things and do not tend to get at these
kinds of subtleties. But in no way did I feel what Toby said meant he would
not have done a Caesar if a Caesar was necessary. At that time he did not think
the woman was in labour, and I did not think that the woman was in labour.
Had that been the case, I certainly would have come in and assessed the size of
the baby myself, and all that kind of thing.*

When I had finished there was a moment of silence. I could feel
the women had understood me, and my lawyers too, but had I
made the men in the room, those on the panel, understand what I
meant? Then John asked me the 'legal' question: *Knowing Dr Fay as
you do, do you think it conceivable that he is the sort of doctor who would let
fatigue interfere with his medical judgement?* I answered, *No, I do not.* Mr
Beaumont asked that: *any corrective reporting should be given the same
prominence.* I thought of how genuine and heartfelt Toby's reply that
morning had been: *We're always tired.* Surely we should not have a
training scheme which left people feeling like that? We as a
profession should be able to organise it better. Part of the problem
at the London was that there was never enough time to deal with
all the interpersonal relationships properly. Maybe, though, that
was a result of our training that men on the whole did not think that
emotions were important. I was glad I had put these ideas into the
enquiry – I hoped that they would be understood. After all, it was
Mr Harvey's use of the word 'sad' which had started off the whole
train of events. The *Guardian* did print my support of Toby and
discussion of the emotions, but *The Times* reported Toby's under-
standably angry reaction. On Sunday, Annabel Ferriman wrote a
very sensitive piece in the *Observer*. At the lunch break two women
came up to me and said that they had found my explanation very
moving. I hoped the panel had.

The Forgotten Charge

In essence, my defence was much the same as that given in June
1985 to the chairman. However, when the AU case had been

discussed (before the baby died) at the Wednesday paediatric meeting, and in Professor Grudzinskas' and Mr Bourne's original criticisms, fetal distress had not been an issue. It *was* a point that I had addressed in my comments to Mr Cumberlege because of Professor Dennis' theory of fetal anoxia when I spoke to him in June and I had obtained evidence from an expert that the CTG did not show evidence of fetal distress.

When I had come back to the labour ward about midday to see Mrs U, I had been angry with the lecturer for not carrying out my clear instructions which included re-examining the woman in two hours and letting me know the result in the theatre. I then quickly examined Mrs U myself, put a catheter into the bladder because I anticipated that we would take her to the theatre then and there, and I did not go all through the partogram or read the notes – as I usually do – but spoke to the midwives about the progress of labour. Then the husband said she had not had the two hours of labour that I had promised them. I felt so badly about not delivering the care that I had promised them that I agreed to let the woman have another two hours of syntocinon-induced contractions as the CTG was reactive – a sign that the baby was in good condition. However, I also got his agreement that if there were decelerations – a hard sign of fetal distress – that he would agree to a Caesarean. I had noted meconium when I examined her, but this I put down to the pressure on the baby, which had entered the pelvis by this stage. (Meconium is a substance in the bowel of a baby which, in a breech presentation, may be forced out by pressure on the baby's abdomen. Sometimes the baby will open its bowels and pass meconium because it becomes distressed in the uterus. This often follows a shortage of oxygen.)

As I was talking to the couple I heard Mr Nysenbaum come in behind me, but when I left the labour ward he was no longer there. Then, as I began to read his note, I saw the words 'ARM – unable to reach buttocks'. ARM means 'artificially rupture the membranes', and in my opinion it should not be done until the presenting part is engaged in the pelvis, otherwise the cord may prolapse and an emergency Caesarean section has to be done to save the baby, as its blood supply is cut off. I was so furious that I stopped reading, turned the page over and wrote my own note. I did not see that Mr Nysenbaum had found meconium at his 8.50 a.m. examination. After the baby became ill and I was going through the notes to see if there was any reason why this should have happened, I finished reading his note and realised that I had missed this alleged sign of fetal distress. However, there were some puzzling inconsistencies. Firstly, if the baby was so distressed as to be passing meconium at 8.50, it seems unlikely that it would have been in such good condition at birth five and a half hours later. Secondly, the liquor round the baby was clear at the time the baby was born, so if the baby was as high as Mr Nysenbaum thought, it should have meant that the baby must have started to pass meconium at the moment he ruptured the membranes – which is possible but not very likely. Thirdly, the CTG, though not of good technical quality in parts, showed accelerations right up to the time the operation was done. Although my registrar thought that the CTG showed type 2 dips (a sign of distress) I thought that what he was seeing were in fact accelerations from the base line (a sign of a non-stressed baby). Lastly, although Mrs U was not thought to be having effective contractions, and although the cervix had not changed much over twelve hours (which would support this), the breech seemed to have descended quite a lot between the 8.50 examination and my examination three and a half hours later.

When John Hendy and I were going through the brief that Brian had prepared so carefully and comprehensively, I asked John how I was going to deal with this issue. He suggested that I might bring it in myself at an appropriate moment. I decided to do this in my examination-in-chief when we reached the decision I took at 12.15 about the AU case: *There is another charge here which nobody has thought of.*

The Times headline on 22 February was 'Savage defends view on labour'; the *Guardian* had 'Savage's feelings clouded judgement', but that referred to my admission that I felt I had let the parents down and had not been firm enough in my advice. Both reports mentioned that I had been angry with the lecturer and had failed to notice the entry, but it seemed understandable. As an obstetrician said to me, 'When I read that in *The Times* I thought, that's terrible, and then I thought back over the years and I know there have been times when I have felt like that.'

After this evidence I had quite long discussions with Mr Harvey and Professor Howie about the management of AU's labour. Then I asked if we could go into camera to talk about the Us' evidence, which we did. We spent over three hours talking about the U case, and by mid-afternoon we reached Ms X.

I felt the day had gone better than expected, but I was worried. Three weeks had gone by and I hadn't even finished my evidence. How would we finish in time?

Day 16. Monday, 26 February

The fourth week opened with John just tying up a few loose ends. Then I asked if I could say something because over the weekend I had been thinking about an interchange I had had with Mr Harvey on the question of *fire brigade obstetrics* when I had pointed out to him that women did not die immediately if they had a post-partum haemorrhage (bleeding after the baby is delivered). At one point he had said, *Think of the obstetricians' coronaries,* and without thinking I had replied, *I don't think we should be planning our obstetric services on the basis of obstetricians' coronaries,* and there had been a burst of spontaneous laughter from the benches. So I thought I needed to emphasise that I was not casual in my approach. Mr Harvey had seemed very attuned to Gordon Bourne when he was giving his evidence, and might tend towards the pessimistic end of the spectrum. I was worried that Mr Harvey might go away with the impression, because of my Third World experience, that I was a bit too relaxed about warning signs. *I am not casual, but I believe in looking at the whole person and not just one thing in isolation.*

The Cross-examination

I turned slightly in my chair away from my lawyers and towards Mr Kennedy as he rose to his feet, his round glasses catching the light. He opened with, *Mrs Savage, when Professor Grudzinskas was appointed, that was the first of January 1983, that he took up his appointment, was it not?* I said, *He came on the fourteenth of January because he went skiing for a fortnight first.* This reply clearly irritated him and set the scene for his cross-examination of me, which was to last for over two days. He asked me sharply, *Why did you think it was important for the committee to know he went skiing? To show he was an idler? Why did it matter that he went skiing?* I said, *That is the way my memory works . . .*

Looking back on it, I think that Mr Kennedy made an error in the way he approached his cross-examination of me. I had always thought of the law as a very dry and unemotional process, but sitting in the waiting room sometimes at Bindmans and observing the other clients – noting how Brian, as well as having this objective assessment of people and their motives which was quite detached and unemotional, was also very sensitive to my need to talk about all aspects of the case, not just the legal ones, and seeing at close quarters how he and John had approached the whole enquiry once it started, I realised that there was a lot of psychology involved. I saw too that the whole planning of the case and how to introduce the evidence and how to cross-examine people was just like the best medicine – approaching the topic as a whole, seeing the person in context. Mr Kennedy had had the opportunity of seeing me questioned by the panel and led through my evidence by John Hendy for three days – and only once had I nearly broken down, when Mr Harvey had asked me if I felt sad.

On another occasion I had responded sharply to Mr Harvey, and that was to do with my feelings about obstetrics being organised for the provider, not for the woman. Having taken note, as he clearly had from his line of questioning, of the events since my suspension, Kennedy could have seen that I was a fighter. If he had been sympathetic and been sensitive to my feelings, I think he might have reduced me to tears, and made a case out for me being emotionally unstable or not up to the stress of the job, or something of that nature.

As it was, his treatment of me was unpleasant. He attacked not only my clinical judgement and decision-making but also me as a person, and his approach converted the atmosphere into that of a criminal court. As the March Bulletin of the Institute of Medical Ethics put it, 'Daily reports of the enquiry proceedings did not always reflect the intense distaste that many who attended felt for the event. That distaste centred on leading counsel for Tower Hamlets who seemed to think that an enquiry into a professional's competence required the same style of advocacy as prosecution for a mass murderer.'

Another aspect of this forceful approach was that it seemed to me that the chairman usually deferred to him if he rose to object to John Hendy's questioning, and for example the fuss made about my inadvertent transgression of the rules of evidence on Day 14 was minor compared with the way that the chairman allowed Mr Kennedy to present evidence outside the terms of reference, for example the first two hours of the professor's evidence on Day 2, and another example is given on Day 18.

The way the case was pursued also perpetuated the personal differences in attitude and approach that underlay the whole affair. It has damaged the relationships between the Tower Hamlets Health Authority and the women in the community of Tower Hamlets who it is meant to serve, and between myself and the GPs and the Division of Obstetrics and Gynaecology. In addition, it added to the unfavourable impression of the profession which this affair has given to many people.

The next two and a half days are not so clear in my mind: the endless slow progress through the case notes, the new allegations, the battle of wits as Mr Kennedy kept on trying to trap me, his manner varying between condescension and irritation with my thoughtful answers. There was a moment of laughter when he produced the copy of my circular letter to the Academic Board of Monday 24 February and asked me if I planned a warlock hunt, which made the *Guardian* headline the next day. There was another moment in the afternoon when he, in response to my comment that Susan Payne had told me that she had gone to sleep during her labour, expressed scepticism that she would remember. I told him that even the grandmothers in the room would remember every detail of their labours, and a murmur of agreement ran through the room.

Day 17. Tuesday, 25 February

Mr Kennedy started with some letters from Professor Ritchie who had been dean, pursuing his point of the previous day about how Gedis had tried to get me to reduce my clinical work. Then he continued with Linda Ganderson, and wasted what seemed like hours following a red herring about my not having seen her at the twenty-eight-week visit – which turned out to be because she was on holiday. I found it hard not to betray my irritation as he slowly worked out all the dates and entries. Mr Harvey spent some time questioning me, and Professor Howie helped me out when I was getting tired.

Then Mr Kennedy began on the AU case, going over and over the notes, for more than five and a half hours. I did not feel confident of having reassured Mr Harvey that I had weighed up the risks. I also hoped that Professor Howie had accepted that, in view of her poor labour pattern, I thought the risk of entrapment of the aftercoming head was negligible after two hours of good contractions. I mentioned that I thought the cause of death was idiopathic thrombocytopenic purpura.

Day 18. Wednesday, 26 February

The *Guardian* headline was 'Stillborn baby's mother not seen often enough', and *The Times* had 'Savage tells why she let mother attempt labour' and quoted my reply: *an understanding through her own body that this baby was not going to come out.*

We continued with the AU case. Mr Kennedy tried to discredit my assessment of the depth of her feeling about avoiding a Caesarean section, using the 1980 notes about her first pregnancy, and how she had accepted the senior registrar's advice then.

Finally we got to Denise Lewis, and Mr Kennedy concentrated on the instructions I gave about inducing her labour as evidence of my inability to communicate. Then he asked me to speculate as to how I would be able to work again at the London Hospital if I was cleared. I did not think that this had anything to do with the panel and appealed to the chairman, but he allowed Mr Kennedy to continue this line of argument. Finally, I lost patience with him. I said, *I am sorry, Mr Kennedy, but I think that you are wasting time . . . I do not think I am incompetent. I think these five cases are not perfectly managed. I have admitted fault at certain points, but beyond that I will not go.* He persisted: *This has arisen out of disharmony in the division, has it not, really?* I looked at him in surprise: *You have said so, Mr Kennedy.* I said I would be happy to compare my practice with my colleagues, but I did not want to speculate about what might happen when the panel reported. John Hendy intervened to suggest that I could be asked about specific assurances. I suggested that an enquiry into the Division of Obstetrics and Gynaecology was what was needed – and perhaps the enquiry panel would like to take that on. There was laughter in the room; both obstetricians threw up their hands in horror, and I heard someone saying 'no'. Finally, Mr Kennedy tried to suggest I could not work with the junior staff. I replied, *If the will to work together is there, there is no reason why we should not have a perfectly satisfactorily functioning department.*

My cross-examination was over. John Hendy took up the last point and drew the panel's attention to my letter to Professor Grudzins-kas of 5 March 1984 where I had urged that the professor find 'three wise persons' to help the department to function more productively. John clarified one or two points, and then my evidence was over. I hoped I had got across the principles of management of these cases, even though the way they were cared for was less than ideal.

My supporters had noticed the other side passing round the *Daily Mirror*, and at the lunch break they bought a copy and passed it to us. We read: 'A new competition: spot the accused!' They had worked out deliveries per session from the figures introduced on 7 February and compared them with the perinatal mortality rates. These showed that I delivered more babies than my colleagues per session but had fewer deaths. 'Clue: the accused consultant is the only one who has ever had a baby!' Although I knew that statistically it was unfair to the others, after the tension of the last week, I found it very funny.

CHAPTER 13

Expert Witnesses for the Defence

I can say without hesitation that if the worst five of my own cases over the period of a year were put under a microscope, it would be possible to create a dossier similar to that of Mrs Savage. I believe the same could be done of every consultant obstetrician that I have ever worked with.

Peter Dunn, Reader in Child Health, Bristol University

Dr Iain Chalmers, Director of the National Perinatal Epidemiology Unit, Oxford: The first of our expert witnesses to give evidence was Dr Iain Chalmers, who decided to train as an epidemiologist after obtaining his MRCOG in 1973. Brian Raymond took him through his evidence, and Mr Kennedy intervened several times to complain that he was 'leading', or that his evidence was 'irrelevant', saying that there was no dispute about differences in practice. I thought there may well not be any differences in theory, but in practice that was the nature of my colleagues' disagreement with me: their apparent lack of tolerance towards a different viewpoint.

Iain made the distinction between 'standard practice' or 'accepted practice' which was what doctors did, but which might not be based on good evidence and gave as an example the stilboestrol story. This synthetic oestrogen was used widely in the USA between the 1950s and late 1960s to treat threatened abortion. Then in 1969 it was found to have caused vaginal cancer in a small proportion of the women born to mothers given this treatment. Yet it had continued to be used and was *accepted* practice. *Acceptable* practice, on the other hand, was that which was based on sound evidence.

Brian asked him whether there was 'unified' practice in relationship to some of the issues in the five cases: investigation and treatment of anaemia, length of second stage, IUGR and Caesarean section. His answers were thoughtful and based on scientific work that had been done, or he admitted the profession's ignorance because of research that had not been done. He also said that one

149

could not make a realistic assessment of competence on the basis of an unrepresentative sample of a person's work.

When Mr Kennedy rose to cross-examine him there was an air of tension and his questions were acid in tone. And they became more so as Iain refused to be drawn into making statements other than those he felt were right, and in his quiet but firm way refused to be led into unscientific argument.

You ought to recognise your own fallacies as scientists is the point really, said Mr Kennedy after the stilboestrol story had been given as an example. Iain replied, *By all means refer to it as science if that is helpful. What I am saying is that there is a need for humility amongst all doctors, including research workers like me, in the light of the record of unintended mistakes that have been made in the past, made in the best faith and with a firm belief that they were doing good by the people who came to them for help, but which nevertheless in the long run turned out to be harmful. What I am saying is that if one wants to protect the patients that come to doctors from those unintended mistakes in future and now, then we must be careful before accepting opinion without evidence.* Mr Kennedy looked at him and asked, *Do you say that is wrong?* And Iain said, *Yes, I do. I say that it is wrong to accept opinion without evidence when people's livelihoods are at stake.* Mr Kennedy looked irritated: *If you are not careful you are making noises like a trade unionist!* This was another moment when our side of the room was united against Mr Kennedy. For him it was so clearly a terrible thing for anyone to be an articulate trade unionist!

There were moments of humour when, for example, Mr Kennedy read out some of the instructions about the induction of Denise Lewis, and Iain said, *You have got a lot more written between your lines than I have got on mine, actually.* There was laughter from behind me, and even the panel members smiled.

Turning to IUGR, Mr Kennedy did his best to trip Iain up. However, Iain said that, firstly, the whole question of how IUGR was defined was confused and, secondly, the evidence that you could use to determine who was at high risk of IUGR was heavy smoking and a previous baby who was growth-retarded, not weight at booking. This contrasted with Professor Dennis's evidence the next day. (We had not anticipated that the prosecution case would take more than a week, and as Iain was due to go abroad on 10 February the prosecution allowed him to appear between two of their witnesses.) As regards scanning, routine ultrasound had been shown to identify more babies who were growth-retarded, but not to have any effect on the outcome of the pregnancy. However, some people wanted to be sure that the intervention once IUGR had been diagnosed did more good than harm.

Mr Kennedy looked more and more displeased as the morning wore on, and finally he said, *But there cannot be any question that the prudent practitioner keeps the matter under lively review.* Iain replied pleasantly, *Oh, I am sure that is right.*

Sarcastically Mr Kennedy ended his cross-examination: *It is nice that we can agree. So, really, at the end of the day what you are telling the committee is this: what can we be certain of in this wicked world?* Iain answered steadily, *I have given you some examples. I would be very happy to go on giving you examples of things where I am certain. What I am saying is that there is an awful lot of uncertainty around, and we need to deal with that in a way that is credible.* In his re-examination Brian Raymond remarked, *That I understand, but to use your own words, the committee and nearly all of us are hamstrung.* His glasses flashing, Kennedy interrupted him again: *That is not a question, that is a speech.*

Afterwards Brian and John said to me that Iain had given me a textbook example of how to respond to cross-examination. He had not lost his temper despite the tone of some of Mr Kennedy's questions. He had stuck to his point and not allowed Mr Kennedy to extrapolate from his replies things which he had not meant, and he had thought carefully about the way he answered. I hoped I would be able to do as well.

Dr Marion Hall, Consultant and Honorary Senior Lecturer, Aberdeen: Marion Hall from Aberdeen was the second of our expert witnesses and took her place at the table on Wednesday 26 February, Day 18, a fortnight later. Mr Kennedy had spent so long pursuing irrelevant points and minuscule details in the notes in an attempt to find something to strengthen his case, that there was considerable pressure of time, as Marion had to be back in Aberdeen on Thursday afternoon. John Hendy therefore took her fairly rapidly through her evidence-in-chief. Brian had prepared statements from all our experts dealing with the original fifty-nine charges, and their overall comments as to whether there was evidence for a finding of incompetence. These were given to the panel members either the night before or when the witness came to give evidence.

Several important points were made. Crude weight was not a risk indicator for IUGR – weight for height was more useful, and Linda Ganderson was not in this risk category. Women's own feelings were important in relation to Caesarean section. Consultants were not expected to be governed by the same arbitrary rules as medical students or doctors at the beginning of their careers. In the case of Susan Payne there was no risk to mother and child. Ms X had been managed perfectly correctly. IUGR was difficult to diagnose, and the criticisms that I should have informed my covering consultant were nonsensical – she had worked out that about ninety women might at any one time be under suspicion of IUGR, although Peter Howie questioned this vigorously. Finally, John read from her statement, *'If asked to advise as to whether Mrs Savage should be reinstated, I can only say that there is no basis at all in the information before me upon which she should even have been suspended, and I have no hesitation in recommending her immediate reinstatement.'* She answered firmly, and some indignation crept into her voice, *Yes, I think it remarkable she was suspended on this basis. If the professor . . . felt that he had problems with his relationship with Mrs Savage in respect of her academic work, then it is entirely proper for him, as he is head of the department, to give her instructions about how to conduct her academic work, but he is less clinically experienced than she is, and it is not part of his duty to look after her clinical competence, and I find it very surprising that the Health Authority should have accepted the cases being dredged up in this way and brought up as evidence of incompetence. I think it has been a quite improper way of conducting proceedings.*

Mr Kennedy rose to his feet – a gleam in his eye, his opening question was hostile in tone – because she had used the word 'dredge' he implied she was not an objective witness. Mr Conlin asked that we went into camera, as he put it to her that the cases had been raised at meetings by the junior staff – which John Hendy rose to dispute.

When we resumed the public session, Marion commented reasonably on the habit Mr Kennedy had of looking directly at the panel when he thought he had made a good point or asked a question, the reply to which he wanted the panel to pay particular attention to. Mr Kennedy replied *I am terribly sorry. I do not mean to be rude.* In her soft Scottish voice, Marion said, *It came across rudely.* Mr Kennedy looked surprised – I suppose he was not used to being challenged about his manner in court. *In that case I apologise now and*

I apologise for the times when I shall offend again. (But not, I thought, for the previous times.)

The next morning Mr Kennedy concentrated almost entirely on the AU case. I found it almost unbearable as he put different questions to Marion, points which I had answered, or, where I had admitted I was at fault, different theoretical possibilities. I could hardly keep quiet. It was worse than being cross-examined myself.

When discussing the point as to whether or not Mrs U was going to return to Bangladesh, which later he stated was a 'footling point', Marion said, *I do not know that it is really very appropriate to ask for a firm commitment of: 'Are you going back to wherever you came from?' at 4 o'clock in the morning. I mean, it would sound like a rather hostile question.* Everybody in the room laughed. *You obviously go in for early discharges in Aberdeen. Surely it is absolutely essential if you are going to take into account the woman may go to Bangladesh?* Marion replied, *No . . . her knowledge of the local population would be that there is a fair degree of movement to and fro . . . if that is quite common, then I think that would have to be taken into account.* Mr Kennedy's own viewpoint came out clearly: *Some of us might have thought there was rather more 'to' than 'fro'. Nowadays an increasing number of people from the Third World are settling and making their homes here, so that the general tendency is that the non-indigenous population of this country is increasing?* The second half of this question was almost lost as the people behind me responded to his 'to than fro' by a low hiss. Mr Kennedy responded to the audience's reaction defensively, *You have only got to shut your eyes and think how many brown faces you saw in England fifteen years ago. The answer was many less than today.* One gained the impression he did not think the change was for the better.

He continued pressing Marion about all sorts of tiny details of the management of the AU case, and his manner was condescending and sceptical by turn. He insisted on using the argument that it took an hour to get a Caesarean done at Mile End, despite my evidence that in an emergency that was not so. He and those of my colleagues who insisted on using the poor anaesthetic service at Mile End to attack me were responsible for the headlines the next day: 'Hospital accused of birth delays' in the *Guardian* and, in *The Times*, 'Hospital "should not deliver babies"'.

Marion Hall had responded to his questions by saying that, *Any labour ward which is not able to respond quickly and do a Caesarean section in fifteen minutes should not be delivering babies,* and to a later statement about the anaesthetic arrangements, *But if it is the case that they are administering epidurals without a live-in anaesthetist, then they should be closing the hospital, or else they should have a live-in anaesthetist.* It really upset me to have Mile End downgraded in the way that Mr Kennedy kept on doing, and I thought that the money being used on this enquiry would have paid the salaries for several years of the four anaesthetic registrars said to be needed to provide a proper service.

Last question: is there anything that you have heard, or that has been put to you that has altered your view about Mrs Savage's competence? Marion replied, *Since coming here, do you mean? Yes.* John waited. There was a pause – then she said strongly, and with some emotion, *No, no. I mean, I have been distressed to hear her being accused of lying, because my impression is that she is honest to a fault.* Mr Kennedy brought us back to the law: *That is nothing in point.* Mr Beaumont agreed: *That is not to do with competence.* Mr Kennedy: *That comes from having a public enquiry.*

I didn't think he had understood the point. It was not the publicity, it was the behaviour of doctors, even if it was being done through their legal mouthpiece, that upset Marion Hall. Was it because she was a woman that she had expressed some emotion? Is this why women are so often seen as a 'problem' in professions like medicine and law?

I thought of Marion ringing her children the evening before to make sure that they had got the supper sorted out, how she was chair of their division, involved in local politics, had got her MD, and as an NHS consultant was more involved in research than many academics I knew. And I echoed the views expressed by one of my supporters. Why can't we have more people like that in obstetrics – direct, caring and yet up-to-date and professional? Why wasn't *she* a professor?

Mr John McGarry, Consultant Obstetrician from Barnstaple: John is above average height, with glasses and slightly curly hair. He never rushes into things, but speaks quietly and slowly. He has a great sense of humour, and told the enquiry panel that, having been a senior lecturer and gone up the academic ladder, having done his professor's work for five years and observed what professors do, he had decided to become an NHS consultant because he liked practical obstetrics and he liked dealing with patients.

Mr Kennedy spent almost a day trying to get him to condemn my management of the AU case, and suggested that he was not impartial because of his comments about some of the 'behind the scenes' behaviour. As the hours went by I saw John, steady as a rock, stone-walling the questions. John's obvious sympathy for women came across strongly, and when Mr Kennedy accused me of misleading the parents by saying the woman would not deliver soon instead of never, he replied, *What she is in the business of doing there is what we all do every day – she is giving the lady some hope.*

His own experience of personally delivering over 150 breech babies vaginally had led him to believe that the risk of entrapment of the aftercoming head was overemphasised in the books, and that if the progress of labour was smooth and descent was steady, the risk was negligible. He shared care in all his cases with GPs and midwives, and said that the relationship between GP and obstetrician was the most important factor in deciding on the pattern of care. Also as he had got older he had become less worried about anaemia and he did not treat it unless it fell below 8 Gms. Neither did he use prophylactic iron and folic acid.

He was an unshakable witness. At the end of the day one of the women said to me, 'We have all decided to go to Barnstaple to have our next babies', and one of my friends, a grandmother, said, 'That includes me – what a lovely man!'

We had not met on Friday 28 February, but the lawyers had agreed both to an extra week and extended hours as everyone wanted to get the enquiry over with.

That weekend I had been really depressed. I did not read the transcripts which came about a week after the evidence and were read through by Brian and John, who took note of points which they had not marked in their own daily notes of the case. When I had asked the BMA legal adviser how long it usually took for the panel to report after a 112 enquiry, he had said two weeks. Even though Brian was sceptical because nobody seemed to know much about this procedure, I had held on to this timing. John Hendy had floated the idea with the chairman when the lawyers and panel met that they could announce the verdict at the end of the enquiry and give the written report later. Mr Beaumont had said that this would be ready for the July or September Health Authority meeting. I could not believe that I would have to wait so long – I turned on the answerphone, I ignored the post which needed answering, the untidy house, and read two novels to cheer myself up and put the whole business out of my mind.

The support group who had maintained a rota of women to attend the enquiry, and had brought the mobile crêche once so mothers with young children could come, had arranged to lobby on what we had thought would be the last day, Friday 7 March, with a disco at Oxford House in Bethnal Green in the evening to celebrate the end. Now we were going to work on the Saturday as well, and thinking about Mr Kennedy's slowness in cross-examination I sometimes wondered if we would get all our witnesses in.

Dr James McGarry, Consultant Obstetrician and Gynaecologist, Southern Hospital, Glasgow: The fifth and last week began. Monday was bitty; Professor Taylor came to give evidence while John McGarry was still being cross-examined. Then Dr James McGarry was called to give evidence. He is a quietly spoken man in his late fifties, with a strong sense of justice. He had written a statement after he had read the affidavits about the way the affair had come into being. The statement was a model of clarity, common sense and fairness, and his responses to the detailed charges reminded me of the respect that my Glaswegian teachers in Nairobi had expressed for him both personally and as someone who had taught them. Because we were so short of time, John was not going through these statements line by line. Dr McGarry spoke with his usual quiet authority. He did not think that this method of analysing five cases out of context was a valid way of assessing competence, and originally had made no comments on the five cases at all in his statement:

> It is suggested that an enquiry will allow debate about the five cases. The prospect is an absurdity. Two entirely different questions will be inextricably confused. The first question, the management of the five cases, will quickly become the management of three cases or even one case and will finally dissolve into conflicting opinions. The second question, that of Mrs Wendy Savage's right to retain her post and to be compensated for the damage done to her reputation by her suspension, will be settled in Mrs Savage's favour in less than five minutes . . .

156

He had written that on 28 October 1985 and now we were in the fifth week of this interminable enquiry. John Hendy asked him, *Do you see anything in any of these cases which would justify her removal from practice as an obstetrician either temporarily or permanently?* Dr McGarry looked up towards the panel and said in a firm voice, *Absolutely not.* Because we were running so short of time, John Hendy concentrated on the most contentious points, one of which was the allegation that my management of Mrs U was dangerous. Dr McGarry spoke of the deep impression that the fear of entrapment of the head had on obstetricians, but added that, *In general I would say that the difference between the size of the fetal trunk and the fetal head is not such that it would be at all common for the baby to be born and the head arrested at the pelvis brim.* On the other hand, he took the view that if a Caesarean is going to be done, the earlier it is done the better, although the problem of women wanting to do things their own way was not one he was familiar with in the Southern General Hospital.

When Mr Kennedy stood up, his voice had taken on a totally different tone. Gently, almost obsequiously he said, *I think it revolts you to be discussing these things in public* – Dr McGarry shook his head – *or offends you. Revolts is too strong a word?* Dr McGarry said in an almost inaudible voice, *No, that is not the nature of my objection.* He answered Mr Kennedy's next few questions briefly with 'yes' or 'no' before we went into private session again.

Then after a short break, Mr Kennedy continued his cross-examination. On and on it went. James McGarry gave his thoughtful answers, like a doctor in an academic forum, and Mr Kennedy, naturally, dissected them to score his legal points. In relation to Susan Payne Dr McGarry said that after two hours he would have done a Caesarean section. I remembered John reminding the panel that it did not matter if the individual obstetrician would not have done something in that particular way – it was a question of whether the practice was within acceptable limits – but then he went on to say: *And the other reason which I hinted at – and it is not necessarily very good science – I think that those of us who tend to be conservative about our use of Caesarean section have got to be careful: we must be aware of getting conservatism a bad name. That is, if you push too far in every instance for what might be achieved safely but on occasion it might turn out badly, then the criticism which would be used against one would be quite strong* . . . My eyes filled with tears – I pushed past Brian and John, meaning to go to our room and have a good cry. As I reached the door I could hear that most people were still in the room drinking tea. I didn't want to cry there – I stood outside, swallowing my tears, out of sight of the panel and the press and the other side.

I kept thinking over the details of the Us' case and of the ordeal that my witnesses were being put through. After about five min-utes – it felt like hours – I went back to my seat. Although I wished that I had done things differently in the U case, I was not going to lose sight of the principle behind the management, that if a woman wants to attempt a vaginal delivery or experience labour I will go along with that, as long as she and the baby are healthy. I will not put the options in such a way that really the woman has no choice.

The Paediatric Evidence

The three paediatricians were very impressive and very different in their approaches. Professor Campbell from Aberdeen was very soberly dressed, solid and understated. He gave evidence first and said that the most likely cause of baby U's death was idiopathic thrombocytopenic purpura (a rare cause of bleeding in the newborn baby due to lack of platelets, cells which help the blood to clot), which I will call ITP for short. Although in response to Professor Howie's question he conceded that a multifactorial cause – that is a tentorial tear and platelet deficiency – was possible, on balance he thought it unlikely. He said that there was no evidence that the baby's death had any relation to what happened during the pregnancy. John Hendy asked on Monday afternoon, 3 March, if the Health Authority would withdraw the charge that my management had caused the death of the baby – which, as he pointed out, had been widely reported. Mr Kennedy said he would have to take instructions about this, but the charge was never withdrawn.

Dr Hey from Newcastle was a complete contrast to Professor Campbell: he wore a roll-necked sweater, a sports jacket and open-toed sandals. He gave his evidence rapidly, almost bubbling over with words, ideas and enthusiasm about his subject. Mr Kennedy, having been very polite to Professor Campbell who does a lot of medico-legal work for the Medical Protection Society, looked at Dr Hey with an air of distaste and leapt upon his use of the word 'wolfed' (in his description of the baby's milk intake) in an effort to throw doubt on his evidence. However, Dr Hey has a thorough grasp of neonatal paediatrics and Mr Kennedy was unable to shake him scientifically. Dr Hey was very careful to say that one could not prove the cause of death, but the balance of probabilities led to it being a lack of platelets as the primary cause, with the most likely reason for this being ITP.

He confirmed what Professor Campbell had not had time to elaborate on, that Baby X had no skull fracture visible on the films.

In the case of Linda Ganderson, Dr Hey told the panel that each obstetrician is likely to have two deaths every three years, which mirrored her case. The only differences were that the notes were of a much higher standard than those he had seen in the Northern Regional Perinatal Survey where most of the cases were completely missed, whereas in Linda's case the IUGR had been picked up, and she had been admitted to hospital.

Peter Dunn, the Reader in neonatal paediatrics at Bristol was heard on Wednesday 5 March, Day 22 of the enquiry. Tall and loose-limbed, he looked too big for the chair at the witnesses' table. He was an excellent witness and, like all our expert witnesses, his vast clinical experience and theoretical knowledge was impressive. He had also discussed the U baby's blood results with the director of his regional blood transfusion service, whereas Gordon Bourne, John Dennis and Gedis Grudzinskas hadn't even discussed them with their local haematologist before accusing me of causing the baby's death. All three of them said ITP was uncommon, occurring in one baby in 5,000. Edmund Hey had reviewed the literature and found that 12 per cent of these babies die, that is about one in 40,000 births. Peter Dunn also said he had seen two cases similar to this in thirty years.

As far as the theory about a tentorial tear was concerned, Peter Dunn saw perhaps, one case a year in Bristol. In Baby U's case, the mild birth asphyxia (found in 25 per cent of babies born by Caesarean section) and the good condition of the baby for twenty-four hours after birth made the diagnosis of this type of tear exceedingly unlikely.

I wondered whether, if we had had a perinatal meeting, a diagnosis of ITP would have been reached. And why was it that we never had enough time for the junior staff or ourselves to go to the library and do a literature search? We must also involve other people – because the haematologist might well have been able to reach this diagnosis, and then the parents would not have had so much suffering.

When John Hendy turned to Baby X, Mr Kennedy rose to his feet and said he had spoken to Dr Harris, the London Hospital paediatrician who had looked after Baby X and Baby U. He had never thought Baby X had had a fracture. I thought of the *New Society* article, headed 'Incompetent health authority': it was all of seventeen months after the birth and into the fifth week of the enquiry before they conceded this. During his evidence we had been given the Baby X notes, and suddenly I saw Ms X's labour CTG. I had a quick look: the transient tachycardia (abnormally rapid heart rate) that had been reported by the midwives at 8 p.m. was there, but the rest of the trace was normal. I handed it to Brian, who gave it to Mr Dibley in the coffee break.

Gordon Stirrat, Professor of Obstetrics and Gynaecology, University of Bristol: Gordon Stirrat is serious and thoughtful; another Scot, he seemed to me to be the same sort of person as Peter Howie. In his evidence-in-chief he did not withdraw from his own position about AU, but had this to say: *I am very aware of the aversion to Caesarean section amongst particularly the Bengali community. We have such a community within Bristol . . . the aversion to Caesarean section goes beyond, in one sense, what we might call reason . . . I can certainly see that that was an important force in the decision to try to achieve vaginal delivery . . . I have a recent example of a Bengali woman under my care . . . She came into my hospital in labour, and was obviously, as time went on, in obstructed labour . . . Progress was not being made, so Caesarean section was counselled, over a lot of resistance, although . . . counselling had taken place beforehand, and the baby actually was fit and well . . . The community midwife . . . reported to me on Friday of last week that she was very concerned about that woman because the husband was now rejecting his wife – she thought the husband was rejecting his wife because she had been a failure . . . the midwife then reminded me of another case . . . again from the same community, and the woman had a Caesarean section for reasons which were absolutely cast-iron . . . That was two years ago. This woman is now in one of our local long-stay mental hospitals, and the psychiatric opinion is that the triggering factor in a woman who was predisposed to this anyway was the Caesarean section and her husband's response to the fact that she had Caesarean section, so two cases have recently been borne in on me in which a proper decision to carry out a Caesarean section has very severe effects in one case and possibly horrifying effects in another, so I am very aware of the problems.*

Gordon Stirrat said he thought the criticisms of the management of Denise Lewis's anaemia were *absurd*, and she did not have severe pre-eclampsia in June. In answer to John's question about my competence in relation to her he replied, *In no way, shape or form can she be described as incompetent in this regard. If it were, I suggest that the majority of obstetricians are similarly incompetent.* In Ms X's case there was no incompetence, and with Linda Ganderson it was regrettable that I had missed her at thirty-six weeks. But on admission, Gordon Stirrat said, *Intervention at that point could have resulted in a live birth.* He looked at the AU traces and confirmed that there was no evidence of fetal distress. Finally . . . *I, really, honestly, reading these notes, found it quite incomprehensible that a claim of incompetence was being made in the context of these five cases . . . one cannot possibly make a diagnosis of incompetence based on one case. If that is the way . . . then questions must be asked about every obstetrician who is practising in this country today. I certainly would not like . . . five cases picked out to be viewed by a tribunal such as this. I would be quite embarrassed.* I looked at Mr Kennedy. He was staring at him with that detached expression.

John went on: *If the management of these cases does demonstrate incompetence, what implications do you see for obstetricians?* Gordon Stirrat replied, *Very, very serious implications for the whole of obstetrics in this country. It would be a decision which would move us very significantly towards the defensive medicine position which we are only too well aware of · from across the Atlantic . . . There is no single body of practice which is agreed within obstetrics in this country, and one has to ask why that is . . . There are basic scientific facts about so many of our practices that are lacking. We are practising on the basis of our training, our experience, such scientific knowledge as is available. If I had to encapsulate my job, it is as a risk assessor.* Mr Kennedy asked a lot of questions, but his heart was not in it.

The Tower Hamlets General Practitioners

Tony Jewell, who is Denise Lewis's GP; Felicity Challoner, who has been a house officer on my firm as part of the East London Vocational Training scheme; and Katy Simmons, who had worked as an SHO with Peter Huntingford, as a locum registrar for me and was now doing her trainee year for general practice at South Poplar Health Centre, gave evidence on Day 23 of the enquiry.

Felicity, obviously a caring doctor, was very quiet, and I found her evidence moving. She said she had never had any difficulty in understanding my instructions and had found no great differences at her level between my practice and that of my colleagues. In cross-examination, Mr Kennedy had modified his tone towards her. In a fatherly manner, he asked her if she remembered any controversial cases from her six months. Two, she replied. He only wanted to know about mine. I was impressed by the candid way in which she explained how she and the senior registrar had not diagnosed a breech in labour. In fact, the baby died soon after birth because it had Potter's syndrome (a congenital abnormality incompatible with life).

Katy Simmons, with her Newcastle accent, slightly off-beat but respectable clothes, was refreshingly frank, caring and alive. She confirmed that there were no difficulties in communication, and said she had learnt more in four months working for me than in all her other obstetrics and gynaecology posts together.

Tony Jewell was another excellent, thoughtful witness. His handling of Denise Lewis's antenatal care, and his reference to her healthy twins seen in his baby clinic showed that he was a better-than-average doctor. He spoke for the GPs and mentioned that his own wife and several other GPs and their partners had chosen me as their obstetrician – hardly a mark of incompetence.

Professor Ron Taylor, United Medical School of St Thomas's Hospital and Guy's Hospital: By the time that Ron Taylor took the stand for the second time on Thursday afternoon, everybody was exhausted. Mr Kennedy, however, was back on fighting form and started off with an attack on Ron's affidavit, in which he had sworn that Professor Grudzinskas had said his first task was to change his senior lecturer. Ron Taylor repeated the advice given to him by Professor Ian Donald when he himself had been appointed – that it would take ten years to get his department the way he wanted. How sad, I thought, that Gedis did not take this advice. Ron's quiet voice, with his slight Liverpool accent, his relaxed position at the table and his humour, lightened the atmosphere. He and one senior registrar looked after 1,000 women a year out of the 3500 delivered at St Thomas's Hospital – so much for Professor Dennis and my impossible workload! His tolerance was so obvious in everything he said, and his clinical experience in particular with reference to vaginal breech delivery came across clearly. He said he would be very happy to have me working in his department, and he ended, *Certainly, I couldn't remotely apply the term 'incompetent' to the handling of these cases.* John asked him: *If the question was 'Is Mrs Savage safe to return to practice tomorrow?' what would your answer be?* Ron's answer: *Yes, certainly.*

Mr Kennedy worked hard, and the phrase 'vaginal delivery at all cost' was used at one point. Ron answered reasonably, despite the tone of some of Mr Kennedy's questions, but we were all glad when the day was over.

Day 24. Friday, 7 March

I went to buy five dozen roses for the Support Group who I knew would be lobbying. I had never had so many flowers in my life, and I thought it was time I gave some back. The shop wrapped them individually and I was nearly late. Everybody was standing outside, including BBC News cameras as I tried to park my son's beat-up Jaguar. I distributed the roses. And then we were inside the chamber for the closing speech for the prosecution. In Kennedy's closing speech I did not recognise myself as this terrible ogre of whom the junior staff were terrified, who could not communicate, and was *convinced of the advantages of vaginal delivery to a point where she subordinates the patient to that wish*; in addition, I was *a crusader with perhaps a sharp temper*, which was one of Kennedy's most memorable criticisms, and a person *with that grave defect of character which is an inability to recognise fault in one's self.* He accused me of lying, of being unable to communicate with the junior staff, and then right at the end he brought up the fact that I had not called Peter Huntingford. The reason that I had not done this was because I thought that he would not be seen as an objective expert witness, having been my professor – and now even this was thrown back at me!

John and Brian were quite pleased, indicating that if the opposition resort to character assassination it means they know they have no case, and I was quite surprised at how detached I felt from this speech. I suppose that if you do not respect a person it does not matter what he or she says and you do not believe that reasonable people are going to be influenced.

As we finished early, I suggested that the panel members visit Mile End. Gedis had another engagement, so I took them round with one of the administration people and the new Mile End midwifery sister. Ironically, in the labour ward we met the midwife who found that Baby U was ill when she came on duty, and on the post-natal ward the sister involved in Susan Payne's first labour. I felt quite sad going round my hospital, but the nurses were glad to see me, and I wanted to be back at work.

Day 25. Saturday, 8 March

It was a beautiful sunny day; it felt like spring, and I hoped this was a good omen. The chamber was packed, as lots of people who worked during the week were now able to come. Mr Badenoch rose, apologised for Mr Kennedy's absence, and brought in another point about competence depending on the consultant's ability to lead a team, i.e. to be a captain.

John Hendy disposed of this later intervention as *legal mumbo-jumbo* and opened his speech with a story about a film in which the hero had bought an Old Bailey kit and found himself, when he had put it together, in the dock in No. 1 court. He invited the panel to tear down the edifice that had been erected over the last five weeks and get back to the atmosphere of a coffee room in a busy hospital. His speech was on a different level from Mr Kennedy's – he defined incompetence, he referred to the various legal definitions, he destroyed all of the new case by reference to evidence in the enquiry using the day, and page and paragraph numbers. I was very impressed by the way he marshalled the evidence together and presented such a good case.

We ate lunch, and afterwards John invited the panel to give us the verdict then and there – and write their reasons at leisure. He presented a letter from the GPs asking for this. I knew that the DHA had also supported a rapid verdict but, although we had the impression that the obstetricians were willing to agree, Mr Beaumont was not. John tried again. The chairman said that they would retire, but if they did not reappear within a minute, we could assume that they had refused our request . . . and then the lawyers were called in to see them.

I felt sorry for Gedis Grudzinskas, alone on the opposite side of the room. His counsel had deserted him, and there was not one of his colleagues with him – as had been the case for most of the five-week enquiry. Apart from the Us' solicitor, only twice had there been a woman on those benches: the wife and an ex-pupil of Mr Badenoch's. I wondered how he felt after five weeks away from his work. He left on his own.

I had got some champagne to celebrate the end of the enquiry, and I went and got the bottle and the glasses. Brian and John came back – they had been offered lukewarm gin and tonic. We all drank to what we felt was a moral victory, and I drank to Brian and John, who had worked so hard for me – and for justice.

That night we went out for a celebratory dinner: the legal team, Luke Zander, and Sam Smith, and their wives, and Sue Hadley and Heather Reid from the support group; Katy Simmons came later; (Felicity Challoner was working for her Diploma in Child Health, and Tony Jewell had another dinner party; Ron Taylor was up in Scotland). We had a great party. It was Brian's idea, and the right thing to do, as the anticlimax of having to wait four months for the result was terrible.

· CHAPTER 14 ·

The Long Wait

'But this second acquittal isn't final either,' said K., turning
away his head in repudiation. 'Of course not,' said the painter.
'The second acquittal is followed by the third arrest, the third
acquittal by the fourth arrest, and so on. That is implied in the
very idea of ostensible acquittal.' K. said nothing. 'Ostensible
acquittal doesn't seem to appeal to you.'

Kafka, *The Trial*

The day after the enquiry ended I flew to Liverpool to open a
Women's Health Bus. It was sad to see the devastation of this
once-thriving city, but the women were terrific. I felt at home in the
informal atmosphere, wearing my dungarees after five weeks in a
tailored tweed suit. Returning to London, it felt strange on the
Monday not to be going to Addison House. Doing something for
long enough can make it begin to feel normal. The atmosphere had
been so intense – reading the transcripts in the evenings – it
became my whole life. I almost missed it! It was the same with my
suspension. Sometimes I felt that *not* practising as a doctor was the
way it was going to be for ever.

I looked at the pile of unanswered mail that had come during the
enquiry. I had started off well, filing it in my 'support' folders and
sending out a standard letter of thanks, but after the first ten days
when the transcripts began coming, I had got behind. It cheered
me re-reading all the letters and I was amazed to find that there
was over £2000 in personal donations to the Appeal Fund. I felt
humbled by the people who, despite living on supplementary
benefit, had written enclosing small sums. I could not let them all
down, but I felt emotionally volatile. Some days I was buoyed up
by the feeling that we had fought the battle well: other days I felt
depressed. The wait seemed interminable.

During the enquiry, Dr Noel Olsen, a community physician in
Hampstead, had been rapidly collecting the 250 signatures needed
to hold an extraordinary general meeting of the Medical Defence
Union to discuss why they had decided not to support me. The
meeting took place on 18 March and the decision was taken that
the MDU would pay my legal costs. I felt very cheered by this but

hoped the public would not think I had been raising money under false pretences. Tony Jewell, the Chairman of the Appeal Fund, put out a press statement which announced Sam Smith's sudden death and stated that the £60,000 raised to pay my legal fees would be banked until I was satisfactorily reinstated. If there was any money left the donors would be contacted.

In March, and after many publishers had expressed an interest, I made the decision to write this book. I had not anticipated how, when I sat down at the Amstrad, I would relive the whole experience. Often I was overtaken by the emotions I had not had time to feel before, and I cried or felt too depressed to write anything for days. I had not thought it would have been so difficult as I had all the documents to hand, but the memories that came flooding back kept on disconcerting me.

Waiting for the Report

On 3 June, Brian wrote to Mr Beaumont pointing out that in order for the report to be considered by the DHA at their meeting on 10 July as promised, it needed to be in our hands by mid-June. The circular gives the accused doctor two weeks to check the first part of the report, the facts, for accuracy, and once this is returned the panel then issue the second part – the findings or, in my case after the 'trial', the 'verdict'. Obviously the DHA members would need time to read and digest this before their meeting to decide about my reinstatement. Mr Beaumont replied on 5 June but gave no date. By mid June, when there was no sign of the report, we asked the Support Group if there was any chance of postponing the march which had been planned too coincide with the DHA meeting. Plans were too far advanced, however, as the posters had been printed and advance publicity was unstoppable.

As the time dragged on we became more and more convinced that we were not going to have the report in time for the meeting. However, a journalist who had spoken to Mr Beaumont told us that the latter had said that having read Part 1 it would be clear what Part 2 was going to be. My answerphone worked overtime, referring the press to Brian, and the pressure mounted as we got to the end of June.

Through the legal grapevine we were given an ongoing progress report on the timing of the report. The first part was finally ready at lunchtime on Wednesday 9th. Brian took the train to Rugby at 1 p.m. to pick it up and I went to the first Dorothy Russell Memorial Lecture at the London Hospital that afternoon. She had been a distinguished neuropathologist, a London Hospital graduate and Professor of Pathology. I forced myself to try and concentrate. At 5 p.m. I rang Brian. 'We've won,' he said and he had already set in motion the contingency plan for a press conference if the report was as clearcut as it had been rumoured to be. I went and joined the neuropathologists, neurologists and neurosurgeons for salmon and strawberries and white wine, but I was too excited to eat and left at 5.45. I rushed to Brian's office to read the report. Brian opened some champagne, and photocopied the first and last parts which we had decided to give out at the press conference the following day. John Hendy called in at about 10 p.m. and had the last glass of champagne. I wondered if all those who talk about the only winners being the lawyers knew how many hours both Brian and John had put in during the enquiry.

Thursday, 10 July 1986

The following morning I drove to the press conference at Queen Mary College Student Union. Although the media had been following the case throughout the whole saga, over the last fortnight interest had reached fever pitch. The Support Group Committee were already there preparing for the evening cabaret planned for after the march and, as we started, with the TV cameras whirring behind their blazing lights, Sue Hadley and Heather Reid presented me with a beautiful bunch of flowers. Brian began with a carefully prepared speech. When had he written it? He must have spent hours on it after we had left his office the previous night. 'The nightmare is over. The attempt to accuse Wendy of incompetence has been shot down in flames. The women of Tower Hamlets will soon have back among them the obstetrician they want.' He had counted up the separate charges, fifty-nine were listed, fifty-five were found to be invalid or insubstantial, and in four instances there were criticisms of my management which did not amount to incompetence.

I had not prepared a speech. I began by thanking all those who had helped and supported me, saying how relieved I was that the panel had cleared me of incompetence. 'I feel I have been vindi-

cated, although I have never said that my work was free of errors.'
The criticisms that were made were all, bar one, accepted by
myself as errors in the comments I gave to the chairman in 1985.
After the press conference various television and radio journalists
asked me to do interviews. We finished about 1 p.m. and I drove to
Whitechapel to put some wine in the refrigerator for after the
march, and then back again for the march itself.

It was a lovely sunny day but not too hot. There were balloons
and babies, women wearing the new badges 'Women need Wendy', several local GPs and Ian Mikardo and Jo Richardson, two of
the MPs who had supported me throughout the long suspension.
Photographers were jostling for position as we started the march
led by Ian Mikardo and myself. It was extraordinary to be at the
front, with all the photographers walking backwards, traffic being
slowed down and hundreds of people with babies and pushchairs
and a band. It both cheered and saddened me, as I saw so many of
my patients amongst them whom I'd not been able to care for all
these months.

The march continued to Vallance Road gardens, where the
police unceremoniously asked the meths drinkers, who were sitting
peacefully in the sun, 'to move on' – the only thing that marred the
day – and everyone sat down and produced picnic teas, bottles of
milk and the kids played on the swings. When the party broke up I
had a small celebration with my sister and other close supporters
before going on to the cabaret at Queen Mary College. It was a
very good party – the feminist groups who entertained us were
amusing and professional and the food from the Punjab cooked by
one of my patients and from Somalia cooked by women from the
Maternity Services Liaison Scheme was delicious. Everyone was
there: Brian and John and their wives, all the members of the
support group, students, and people from the trades council and
local council, journalists and general practitioners, midwives and
nurses, women who had had babies and those who had been
gynaecological patients of mine – it was a friendly and happy
occasion and I felt welcomed back into the community.

The newspapers all carried the story the next day, many placing
it on the front page. It was interesting to see how seriously the
media had taken the whole struggle which could so easily have
been reduced, as one headline put it, to a 'Savage Squabble'.

The Second Part of the Report

Over the weekend Brian and I went through the report, checking it carefully. We met on Tuesday to compare notes and on Wednesday 16 July the few typing errors and interpretations about which we differed were delivered to Mr Beaumont.

On 20 July, the *Observer* carried an article, 'Savage faces ban on comeback'. It suggested that the second part of the report would 'make circumspect comments about the case which would embarrass the Health Authority and, unexpectedly, Mrs Savage herself'. Brian had replied to this firmly: 'Members of the panel would be stepping outside their powers if they made any comments. If the Health Authority fail to reinstate Mrs Savage they will be punishing the innocent victim and rewarding those who made false accusations against her.' Once again the rumour and gossip circuit seemed to have been working overtime and when I was interviewed for the Today programme on the Tuesday I could deduce from the questions I was asked what a panel member had been saying to the press 'off-record'.

On Monday 21 July Brian heard from Mr Beaumont that the second part of the report, including our copy, had been sent to the DHA on Saturday 19 July. I went over to the district offices to collect it. I knocked on the door of Mr Alway, the new general manager. Sitting in the room were Mr Cumberlege, Mr Alway at his desk, and another official. I explained why I had come; Mr Cumberlege said he had been called from a 'luncheon engagement' to see the report, which he was just reading. Mr Alway said I could have a copy, and I sat down to read it. No incompetence, so no disciplinary action. Relief flooded through me. However, because of the implications for patient care the panel had made some observations:

10.2 These matters of concern are referred to in part one of the report. In broad terms they can be categorised as
a) poor working relationships between Mrs Savage and some other consultants.
b) poor communication between medical staff.
c) unsatisfactory cross-cover arrangements between obstetric consultants.
10.3 We do not seek to apportion responsibility for those matters in any way. We recognise and respect the genuine differences of

opinion and deeply held views of the individual consultants. A practical solution would be to separate the obstetric units at Whitechapel and Mile End. This could be achieved by Mrs Savage and another consultant (perhaps a new appointment) being responsible for Mile End, whilst the other present obstetric consultants would be responsible for Whitechapel.

10.4 We also recommend that when unfamiliar methods of management are being employed, the consultant concerned should be closely and personally involved at all stages.

Mr Alway told me that the DHA would release this to the press the following day at 2 p.m. Mr Cumberlege confirmed that a special DHA meeting would take place on Thursday 24 July. I left – it seemed unreal – a certificate of competence at last. I went to see a senior member of the hospital consultant staff. 'We are back to where we were in April 1985,' he said. I answered 'except £250,000 poorer, and my patients deprived of my services for all that time'. I felt depressed. Although we had won, the battle would continue. I had admitted mistakes, but it seemed it was too much to expect that anyone else would publicly. I could see the reluctance to face the issues that had caused this debacle. A satisfactory result, justice had been done, banish the 'odd-one-out' to Mile End. I could see that this was a pragmatic solution, but was it right that this small group of men could get away with the damage that they had caused? The last hurdle lay ahead: would the DHA recommend my reinstatement? It seemed a foregone conclusion, but after the last fifteen months I would not believe it until I heard it.

The Health Authority brought out the result on Wednesday, the day of the Royal Wedding. It was duly reported that Mr Cumberlege was going to propose that I be reinstated, and ask the Authority to ratify a proposal, which had been discussed at a previous meeting, that an advisory panel of eminent persons be set up to consider the observations of the panel.

That afternoon Brian and I went to see Mr Alway and the new solicitor representing the North East Thames Region. We read the press release. I was pleased about the recommendation for reinstatement, but slightly alarmed at yet another panel of enquiry. After the meeting we wrote a letter to the DHA making it crystal clear that I was not prepared to remain suspended indefinitely whilst another panel decided how to get the obstetricians in Tower Hamlets to work together.

The Authority met the following day at 4.30 p.m. We had arranged with Mr Alway that we would wait in my office in Walden Street where we would be telephoned once the result was known. The call came at 6.15. Brian and I walked round the back of the London Hospital and in the side door to avoid any lurking cameras. Mr Alway came and told us the good news. The Health Authority had voted unanimously to reinstate me. The enquiry panel had been agreed: Dame Alison Munro who had chaired the Maternity Care in Action DHSS working party, a representative from the RCOG, and Mr Alway himself. They would prepare a report for the DHA meeting on 11 September 1986 which would enable me to be back at work by mid-September. Brian made some arrangements about the press conference which was scheduled for 7.30 that night. I thanked Mr Alway and we left, almost unable to take it in that it was finally over. At the same time there was a feeling of unreality – was it really over? – and an awareness that there was still another panel to convince.

Back in my office I did a phone-in programme and then we set off for the press conference. It had already started and Mr Cumberlege was answering questions, with Mr Alway on his left and Jean Richards on his right. Mr Cumberlege saw me standing at the back, 'Do come and sit down, Mrs Savage, I do hate to see a woman standing.' I could feel the women behind me almost ready to burst into shouts of rage. I sat down about a yard from Jean Richards and observed the session. Someone asked Mr Cumberlege if he thought it had been right to suspend me; he mentioned the ridigity of the procedure, how in two two-hour meetings he had made the decision and weighed things in the balance. Had he expected the public support? Yes, he had taken that into consideration. I looked at him in disbelief.

The press were pretty kind to Mr Cumberlege, I thought. Amongst other things he said that Mr Bourne had no connection with Tower Hamlets – technically true, but what about our joint Academic Department which meant I met regularly with him, what about his training of the professor and the lecturer? Could he not have said that with hindsight it might have been better to consult someone less closely connected? Someone asked about the proposal that I work at Mile End and how this departed from the district's plan; 'India was partitioned in 1947,' he replied. A gasp of amazement rose from the supporters in the back of the room.

Linda Lewis, a BBC reporter, asked why he had refused to appear in front of the TV cameras and he explained that he didn't like the way he looked on the television screen. He continued: 'I prefer steam radio.'

Mr Cumberlege drew the press conference to a close and we moved to another room where Mr Alway had agreed to do a TV interview. Brian and I then answered questions. I said how delighted I was with the result, that even if the response from the public had not surprised Mr Cumberlege it had astounded and impressed me, and that I thought it a sad comment that after being a chairman of various boards for thirty years in the NHS it had taken an enquiry costing an estimated £250,000 to convince him that doctors held different opinions. Brian spoke strongly: 'The decision that Mrs Savage is not incompetent clearly has implications for those who said she was. They have their consciences to examine.' Radio 4 and LBC then wanted interviews and finally about 9.30 it was over. We went to a pub opposite the London Hospital where we celebrated somewhat more modestly than at the end of the enquiry.

The next day Brian and I made an appointment to discuss our submission to the Munro enquiry panel. The battle had been won, but the terms of the peace had yet to be agreed. The Governors of the London Hospital Medical College had an emergency meeting, and the Dean Elect wrote to me on 28 July suggesting I work at Mile End, thus avoiding the issue. The situation reminded me of the article by Anthony Clare, Professor of Psychological Medicine at Bart's in the *Daily Telegraph* on 12 July: 'Throughout all this the London Hospital Medical College stood aloof, although one of its professors was publicly accusing one of its senior lecturers of incompetence. A better example of the current spinelessness of much of academic medicine would be hard to find.' He ends his article: 'the hushed silence of the medical profession in the face of such a lamentable farce (with one or two admirable exceptions) was one of the most depressing aspects of a most depressing tale. But if there is a moral and I suspect there are a few, it is that if doctors yield their right to regulate themselves up to administrators, managers and lawyers, then such claim as they have to be a profession disappears. And they should not be surprised if the dignity, the standing and the respect that a profession commands disappears with it.'

· CHAPTER 15 ·
Birth and Power

The public has the right to expect a great deal of the medical profession in relation to our standards of professional conduct and practice. We have always set very high standards for ourselves and must surely continue to do so, knowing as we do how easily this vital public trust, which we value so highly, can be damaged.

Sir John Walton, General Medical Council report, 1984

The fifteen months of my suspension from my post at the London Hospital and the subsequent enquiry has been a terrible waste of NHS funds. It has damaged relationships between the GPs and obstetricians in Tower Hamlets and it has reduced, both at the service level and personally, choice for women in the district, especially those women who want a woman obstetrician and gynaecologist. It has prevented over a hundred medical students from being taught by a woman with a different approach to the subject, and it has damaged the reputation of the London Hospital, its Medical College and those doctors involved. Yet I do not accept 'the only winners have been the lawyers'.

The debate about obstetric care has been widened and women have had the opportunity to see that obstetricians can hold radically different views about how childbirth is managed. The women in Tower Hamlets have found a voice and a way of putting their views forward. The three major childbirth consumer organisations, the NCT, AIMS and Maternity Alliance have come together publicly for the first time and an ongoing 'think tank' on maternity care is going forward. Midwives have been strengthened in their battle to regain professional autonomy. Chairmen of Regional Health Authorities have started moves to change the disciplinary procedures for doctors, and some individual doctors have begun to fight against their demoralising, long drawn-out and expensive suspensions.

There are at least six important issues arising from my suspension:

■ Birth and Power – who controls childbirth?

- What kind of services do women want – and who is going to decide on the kind of care that is offered to them?
- Accountability – of the District Health Authority and of doctors.
- Incompetence – how is it defined? How does one measure it?
- Disciplinary procedures for doctors in the NHS – can they be improved?
- Academic freedom and the role of professors and senior lecturers.

- The issue of birth and power is one which arouses strong emotions, because birth is a profoundly moving experience for all those who participate in the drama, whether as the person who should be the central point of the whole event, the woman, or the person who should be in a supporting role, the midwife or doctor.

Birth arouses primitive and elemental feelings within us, reawakens unconscious or conscious memories in connection with our own beginnings and those of our siblings. It reminds us of death as well as life, and the awareness of the tragedies which do still occur is not far from the surface.

Throughout history women have controlled birth in most cultures, and still do in many parts of the Third World. In the developed world men-midwives began to take over the control of birth in the eighteenth century. In the twentieth century the power of the obstetrician has risen to unprecedented heights. In the last forty years we have seen in this country a complete take-over of the whole process of birth by obstetricians, 88 per cent of whom are men at consultant level, where hospital policies are dictated. Only 1 per cent of women still have their babies at home, whereas before the Health Service almost half of all women delivered in their own homes. Midwives were responsible for the care of the majority of women and worked independently.

This major change in childbirth patterns in society has been followed by increased medicalisation of birth and rising rates of intervention, without good scientific evidence that these high rates are necessary. It is true that childbirth is safer than ever before, and that a woman is more likely to have a live baby than ever before, but the relationship between these improvements and many of the changes that have taken place in the 'management' of childbirth have not been properly evaluated and in particular, the fall in perinatal mortality is probably as much related to improved living standards, and easier access to contraception and abortion, as to neonatal intensive care and high technology in obstetrics – although for an individual woman these may make all the difference between a successful outcome and losing her baby.

In particular, antenatal care has not been subjected to rigorous analysis, and yet it has been accepted as essential to a good outcome. Fetal monitoring became widespread before its effectiveness was tested by a valid trial; induction of labour reached 40 per cent a decade ago, with no evidence that this high rate was necessary or even useful. And now the seemingly inexorable rise in the rate of delivery by Caesarean section is justified by some obstetricians for the sake of the baby, but although in some instances this is valid, in others the benefit is not proven.

Although obstetricians justify their takeover of birth by reference to the improved outlook for mother and baby, and although there have been many advances for which women are grateful, there are still a large number of situations about which doctors lack adequate information to say which is the best course of action. My philosophy, in which I am not alone, of involving the woman in the decisions about her care, means that the obstetrician must relinquish some power. Accepting that the woman should have control over her own fertility by means of access to contraception and abortion on her terms, not those of the medical profession, and understanding that the woman should have choice about the way her pregnancy and labour is conducted, seems to be deeply threatening to some obstetricians – of both sexes. Such demands also challenge that power which has been based on a way of looking at evidence which proves the virtues of hospital or interventionist obstetric care over the traditional home-based, non-interventionist practice of midwives.

Although women may not have analysed their dissatisfaction with the care that they have received during childbirth, many hundreds have responded to my suspension by writing letters which show clearly that they do see this issue as a struggle for the control of birth. Women – and the feminist movement – must involve themselves in this battle before we reach the situation in the USA where midwifery is illegal in most states, and where over 24 per cent of women were delivered by Caesarean section in 1985.

■ What kind of services do women want and who is going to

decide on the kind of care that is offered to them? This is part of the wider issue about the way services are provided in the NHS: whether doctors and nurses are the best people to make decisions about what patients need and want, or whether administrators, either as non-practising doctors or as general managers with no medical background, should decide on grounds of efficiency alone. Sometimes when one looks at the cuts one feels that the ultimate hospital, as far as some planners are concerned, would be one which had no patients and thus required no revenue to run it!

My own feeling is that there needs to be a partnership between the consumers and the providers, both medical and administrative. It is too easy for the professionals to become distant from the reality of patients' feelings. For example, doctors and midwives feel at home in hospitals, the surroundings are familiar, we know all the people, we have the pleasure and satisfaction of having accomplished worthwhile work in the building, and it is hard for us to see the place as an outsider does, frighteningly impersonal, overlarge, filled with remote people in a rush – and often associated with unhappy memories of illness or death. The routine, the forms, the technology may make some people feel secure but others feel lost and depersonalised – the very size overwhelms them. In this frame of mind understanding explanations becomes difficult, and the patient is acutely sensitive to attitudes and the way things are said and done.

There are two reasons why this debate is particularly contentious in obstetrics and gynaecology. Firstly, the majority of consultants are men, whereas the consumers are all women. Secondly, many of these women are not ill, they are seeking help and advice about how to avoid pregnancy, or how to get pregnant, how to obtain an abortion or what is best for themselves and the baby if they decide to embark on a pregnancy. Pregnancy is not an illness; it is a very important part of a couple's life together or a woman's life if she decides to go it alone. Women need help to achieve the kind of birth they want – about which many of them, even young women or those with little formal education, often have strong views. The role of the doctor is that of a counsellor rather than that of an authoritarian, trained professional, and this is very hard for some doctors to accept – especially the majority of male obstetricians.

This issue – of who decides on the type of care that a woman gets, the place that she delivers, the importance of her own views – has recurred over and over again in the letters that I have had from women. I think that obstetricians have to take a hard look at the way they are delivering services to women, and join with them in planning for the future so that women have more say, and sterile confrontation is avoided.

■ The third issue is that of accountability. How is it possible that the Chairman of the Health Authority and a handful of doctors could set in motion an enquiry costing an estimated £250,000 at a time when the impoverished district of Tower Hamlets is cutting beds and services? To whom is the Chairman of the District Health Authority accountable? To the people of Tower Hamlets? To the DHSS? To the North East Thames Regional Health Authority? To anyone? The Early Day Motion calling for his resignation was signed by over a hundred MPs in the fortnight between the publication of the first part of the report on 10 July and when Parliament rose on the 25th, but at the press conference on 24 July Francis Cumberlege seemed satisfied with his performance in this matter. He expressed no regret over the cost of the enquiry, nor the damage done to services.

To whom are the rest of the members of the DHA accountable? To the people of Tower Hamlets? To the bodies of whom they are nominees, but not representatives, i.e. the University of London, the Regional Health Authority, the London Borough of Tower Hamlets? The Local Medical Committee of GPs, the Medical Council of the London Hospital, or to none of these bodies? The whole system seems to lack any mechanism for assessing the performance of a Health Authority except in one way – can they keep within their budget?

To whom are hospital consultants accountable for the quality and organisation of their services? To the new General Managers? To the DHA? To the DHSS? To the GMC? To their patients or to no one except themselves? As medicine is a self-regulating profession, in which, quite rightly, clinical autonomy is jealously guarded so that doctors have the right to decide what kind of treatment is best for an individual patient, to whom are doctors accountable – their professional colleagues as represented by the various Royal Colleges?

■ How does one define incompetence in a specialty like obstetrics where there is a wide spectrum of opinion about the best way to look after pregnant women? The legal definition which John Hendy adopted, based on the 1974 NHS reorganisation, was that if the management lay 'within the broad limits of acceptable medical practice' the action could not be said to be evidence of incompetence. Secondly, even if an action was outside these broad limits there had to be more than one deviation. Incompetence must be a continuing state not an isolated event. But what is acceptable practice as far as the professional is concerned? Does this differ from what women think is acceptable practice? Is there good scientific evidence for many of the things that we do in obstetrics – indeed in all branches of medicine? How much of *accepted* practice (based on opinion and current working methods) is *acceptable* practice, which should, as Iain Chalmers said in his evidence at the enquiry, be based on good scientific evidence?

■ Then there is the question of disciplinary procedures for doctors working as consultants in the NHS. Naturally there has to be a mechanism for dealing with doctors who cannot fulfil their duties because of mental or physical illness, dependence on drugs or alcohol, or who abuse their position in relation to patients either emotionally or sexually. Some of these matters can be dealt with through the GMC, and the doctor usually continues to practise until his or her case has been heard.

Occasionally a doctor may be appointed who has not been properly trained, or he or she may become incompetent for one of the reasons listed above. Clearly, for the protection of patients, this person cannot be allowed to practise if he or she is unfit to do so, and suspension is sometimes used as an emergency measure to allow time for the responsible administrative doctor to assess the situation. There is only implied power to suspend, not a well-defined procedure in any of the regulations relating to the employment of consultants.

The procedure used to investigate doctors in whom professional misconduct is suspected, HM (61) 112 is virtually unchanged from the 1951 circular drawn up three years after the Health Service began. It is expensive and time-consuming, and although suspension is not part of the HM (61) 112 procedure, and the Beaumont Panel stated that 'it was not within their terms of reference', it appears that in practice suspension is frequently used concurrently, which is damaging to the doctor, deprives the NHS of his or her services and adds to the expense if a locum is employed.

HM (61)112 does not conform to modern employment law, in which if an employee is at fault he or she must be warned verbally and then in writing. In this case the accused doctor is not told that there is any doubt about him or her until a *prima facie* case has been established to the satisfaction of the Chairman of the Health Authority, who is usually a lay person. It gives no guidance on how to gather evidence or how to obtain expert independent medical advice in the case of incompetence, or how widely the chairman should consult before taking any action. Usually the enquiry is held in private and the 'confidentiality' which is maintained in public allows gossip to thrive and thus damage the doctor's reputation even if he or she is later exonerated by any enquiry.

■ Lastly, there is the issue of academic freedom and the position of senior lecturers within the medical schools. In private many academics will recount the difficulties that they have had with their professors and this, in addition to the uncertainty about academic salaries and poor fringe benefits, makes many doctors who would be good academics choose NHS contracts and greater independence. In time this is bound to lead to poorer training of our medical students and a lowering of standards of doctors. This is an issue that should concern the universities, who cannot pass all the responsibility for standards to the medical schools while retaining all the pomp and status for themselves.

Academic freedom, the right to express opinions, is necessary if we are going to train doctors who can think; and the silence of so many makes the outspoken support of Professor Taylor, Luke Zander and Iain Chalmers, as well as the expert evidence given by those who undertook the unpleasant task of appearing at the enquiry, especially noteworthy.

Many of the letters I have received, as well as the medical and lay press articles and radio and TV programmes, have mentioned one or more of these issues and I think the public debate which followed my suspension has already had positive effects.

The Future

If the dissatisfaction with the way maternity services are provided is to be overcome it is important that obstetricians, midwives and women meet together to discuss how best to use resources and what women want. Their conclusions must then be backed up by research.

The establishment of a study group by the RCOG might enable women to voice their requests in a forum which could lead to change throughout the country, but it needs to be supported by obstetricians as well.

Midwives need to organise and regain their professional autonomy, and take over more of the normal pregnancies and labours. This would please women, especially those with a religious objection to male doctors, and would improve the job satisfaction for midwives. This would also give the obstetrician more time to evaluate what she or he is doing and more time would be spent teaching the junior staff, in particular on the labour ward.

Women need to be more involved in planning local services and they also need to put their requests in a form that administrators can understand. It is a positive gain in Tower Hamlets that the Support Group have started looking forward and are producing a Women's Health Charter which will be presented to the DHA when it is finished.

Changes need to be made in the statutes relating to the appointment of consultants and the way that Health Authorities are formed to increase the representation of consumers. The present system is not democratic and as far as consultant posts are concerned, the influence of a few people, often nearly at the age of retirement, means that the present system is perpetuated.

Incompetence is not a major problem amongst doctors practising in Britain as the training process is rigorous but also fairly personal. But how *are* doctors taught about assessment in medico-legal cases? Is this an area in which a regular practical session could be provided by the RCOG on the steps necessary to write a report, on what evidence is needed and in what circumstances doctors should agree to do this task, and on the need to understand the breadth of medical opinion. Here some basic legal knowledge could be learned before rather than in the course of a case.

Disciplinary procedures for hospital consultants need to be

re-examined by the medical profession in conjunction with experts in employment law. The defence organisations should re-examine the way in which they advise doctors in dispute and see if a better system could be devised.

The medical profession also needs to look at its institutions, and see whether by sharing the power and responsibility, a broader band of doctors would take on the burdens of committee work, examinations, medico-legal work, postgraduate education and other administrative tasks. This would allow those at the top to think and respond to situations such as my suspension, and the incredible waste of public money which followed it. Doctors in senior positions, by ignoring the outcry from their GP colleagues and my patients, despite their appreciation of the injustice of this act and their suspicion that I was not guilty, have threatened the concept of the profession as a self-regulating one. We need to find a way to be more honest and less bureaucratic.

I hope that this book, by adding to knowledge of this whole affair, will help us to go forward and make changes which will be of benefit to both women and the medical profession. Ultimately these issues affect everybody, because the way a society deals with birth affects the whole fabric of that society and sets the scene for the next generation.

· APPENDIX I ·

Particulars of Case

1. *Susan Payne*

1. If the normal treatment for slow or no progress during the second stage of labour in a breech presentation in a prima gravida, namely Caesarean section, was not to be pursued, then a consultant assessment within two hours of the commencement of the second stage of labour should have been undertaken with subsequent consultant assessment and direction being provided personally.

2. Syntocinon should not have been used to augment the second stage of labour.

3. (i) Mrs Savage should not have made a judgement on the telephone that the diagnosis of full dilatation was wrong in the absence of clinical observations of her own to support this disagreement with the reported findings of those on the ward;

(ii) If Mrs Savage did not trust the combined judgement of her juniors, and/or if (as she says in her comments, page 23 (c)), the registrar was to her an unknown quantity, she should not have left matters in that registrar's hands, in particular when disputing the diagnosis, without herself attending.

4. The second stage of labour was allowed to continue for an inordinately long time, namely over 8 hours, in particular having regard to the footling breech in a prima gravida.

5. Mrs Savage's course of management in this case was idiosyncratic, quite outside the limits of normal management, and potentially hazardous to the unborn child.

6. By her assertion that the successful outcome proves her assessment of risk to have been correct, Mrs Savage:

(i) demonstrates a lack of insight into the potential for danger which was inherent in her management, and

(ii) propounds an approach to obstetrics which allows risk taking judged ex post facto by fortunate result.

2. Linda Ganderson

1. This patient was unsuitable for continuation of shared care once growth retardation was suspected. Mrs Savage continued the shared care notwithstanding this suspicion.

2. At 30 weeks gestation intra-uterine growth retardation should have been recognised as the probable diagnosis, but was not.

3. IGR [IUGR] having been so recognised, the patient should have been admitted to hospital for full investigation and inpatient treatment at 30 weeks, namely on 27 February, or at the latest on 12 March 1984, on both of which dates Mrs Savage saw her.

4. The patient was referred back to the sharing GP on 12 March 1984 with Mrs Savage's reference to 'possible' IGR [IUGR] and/or 'wrong dates'. In the premises, the GP was inadequately informed and Mrs Savage delegated to the GP assessment and decision-making which was properly Mrs Savage's responsibility and for which the GP had not the necessary level of training or expertise, as Mrs Savage well knew.

5. Having thus referred the patient back to the GP, Mrs Savage failed to ensure that the patient's progress was monitored expertly and adequately, so compounding the errors above referred to, with the result that the patient was not thereafter seen by Mrs Savage and/or hospital specialist staff for 4 weeks and was not admitted until 18 April 1984.

6. At the time when the patient was admitted on 18 April the junior staff and covering consultant had not been adequately informed by Mrs Savage and/or by the GP with whom Mrs Savage shared the patient's care as to the fact of severe growth retardation and weight loss.

7. The severity of growth retardation was not recognised by Mrs Savage and/or the GP with whom she shared the care of this patient, and their determination to continue this inappropriate management unnecessarily prejudiced the outcome.

3. AU

1. (i) A purported 'trial of labour' was ordained by Mrs Savage and attempted when there were known contraindications which taken singly, but more importantly together, should have altogether precluded any such attempt;

(ii) In the light of all the known contraindications to 'trial of labour', and the attendant risks, it was an improper exercise of Mrs Savage's specialist obstetric role to opt to use 'two hours of good labour . . . to show her that she was not going to be able to deliver vaginally'. (Mrs Savage's comments, page 20 at (e)).

2. (i) The known history of the patient should have compelled an early decision, made in advance of the onset of labour, that there must be an elective Caesarean section as the only safe course;

(ii) In the absence of the decision for elective section, a section should have been performed very much earlier in the course of labour and by 4.00 a.m. at the latest;

(iii) Mrs Savage compounded the dangers inherent in the failure to decide on elective section, and non-performance of timely section during labour, by administering syntocinon (a potentially dangerous drug used for the purpose of strengthening uterine contractions) when she did not herself believe that the baby could safely be delivered vaginally;

(iv) Giving instructions to continue syntocinon but 'to watch the fetal heart carefully and perform immediately Caesarean section if deceleration continued to occur' Mrs Savage failed to ensure such immediate Caesarean section, despite decelerations continuing to occur, until 1.20 p.m. and did not do the section herself, but should have done.

3. (i) The necessary discussion and explanation of the need for elective section should have, but did not, take place well in advance of the onset of labour and should have included, but did not, clear advice about the necessity for that course in the interests of mother and child outweighing the natural preference of the parents for normal labour and vaginal delivery;

(ii) Having failed to discuss and recommend elective section at the early stages of the pregnancy and to make all reasonable efforts to secure informed agreement thereto, elective Caesarean section should have been recommended at the stage in late pregnancy when the fetal lie was found to be unstable with the baby presenting by breech in a patient with a Caesarean scar whose earlier Caesarean had been carried out for disproportion and whose baby Mrs Savage now estimated to be larger than that of the first pregnancy (all of which matters should have been explained);

(iii) The discussion process between the consultant team and the parents whereby the parents ought to have been enabled to participate in, understand and jointly agree the likely necessity for intervention was delayed and inadequate, with the result that the parents were not in a position during labour to make an informed decision;

(iv) The parents' expressed wish, following Mrs Savage's examination of the patient at 12.15 p.m., to have 'another couple of hours effort towards vaginal delivery' should not have been encouraged but should have been the subject of clear warnings as to the known dangers.

4. (i) Syntocinon augmentation was contraindicated but commenced on Mrs Savage's instructions at 9.30 a.m.;

(ii) Whatever the alleged reasons for commencing syntocinon it should not have been continued after Mrs Savage's examination of the patient at 12.15 p.m.;

(iii) Knowing, as she did, that the patient had received epidural anaesthesia and that syntocinon had been commenced, she ordered the drug administration to continue as aforesaid, despite her own allegedly clear instructions about the management of labour given to the juniors and her own express view that – 'epidural is contraindicated in a woman with a uterine scar in which syntocinon is given' – Mrs Savage's comments, page 18 (b).

5. Mrs Savage disregarded at the time, and continues to disregard in her comments on the case, the conclusive evidence of pelvic disproportion.

6. Mrs Savage delayed the decision to undertake emergency Caesarean section notwithstanding her knowledge that, by reason of the geography and organisation of the hospital facilities, there was a predictable delay

between any decision to do a section and its performance of up to 45 minutes.

7. Mrs Savage, having embarked on a course of management which was wholly outside normally accepted practice and carrying with it well known attendant risks, should have been, but was not, personally involved in the important later and more dangerous stages.

8. By her irrational management and continuing failure to appreciate and act appropriately upon a manifestly deteriorating situation throughout the progress of labour, Mrs Savage instigated management which resulted in prolonged and strong uterine contractions in the presence of disproportion and thus, on the balance of probabilities, caused the baby's death or alternatively contributed to the fatal outcome.

4. Denise Lewis

1. Shared care with the GP was inappropriate for this abnormal pregnancy with a known potential for the development of complications.

2. (i) Having regard to the patient's previous history of anaemia and the fact of multiple pregnancy, the development of anaemia was not investigated satisfactorily or early enough;

(ii) Having decided against prophylaxis against predictable anaemia, Mrs Savage failed to inform her covering colleague, Mr Oram, of the potential problem.

3. When iron injections were administered in late May 1984 it was too late to be effective by the time of delivery.

4. (i) Despite severe pre-eclampsia, Mrs Savage decided upon induction in the presence of twin breeches which was a wrong decision;

(ii) Caesarean section should have been carried out electively.

5. (i) Mrs Savage gave instructions at 6.30 a.m. that induction of labour should commence 'that day' on the basis of incomplete and/or inadequate assessment of the patient's true condition;

(ii) Mrs Savage acted as aforesaid notwithstanding her contention made in her comments at page 13(h) that, had she assessed the woman vaginally herself, she would not have induced her with an unfavourable cervix and with a breech 4 cm above the spine.

6. Induction having been decided upon, it was continued for 11 hours which was much too long, in particular having regard to her own awareness that the breech was high.

7. (i) In the light of all the known features of this lady's pregnancy and labour and her previous history, this was a high risk pregnancy. In the circumstances, Mrs Savage:

(a) did not adequately brief her junior staff;

(b) did not ensure her own regular and complete information on progress by telephone or otherwise;

(c) was absent when her own idiosyncratic plan for management dictated that she should be present herself to carry that plan into effect.

(ii) Mrs Savage absented herself as above without ensuring appropriate consultant cover and without informing her consultant colleague that he was indeed required to cover this serious problem case in circumstances where she had provided for her juniors an inappropriate, confusing, and potentially dangerous plan of management.

8. In the light of the known history of this pregnancy and labour, Mrs Savage should acknowledge, but persists in her refusal to acknowledge, that a potentially dangerous condition of pre-eclampsia was present and required immediate steps to effect delivery which were not taken.

9. In the premises Mrs Savage is at fault in seeking by her comments to lay blame at the door of her colleagues and juniors.

5. X

1. A trial of labour was the appropriate management for this teenage prima gravida of short stature (4 ft 10 ins) who had sought late termination, but the procedure followed was not a trial of labour.

2. Notwithstanding that, after 11 hours in the labour ward, the cervix was 5–6 cms dilated, and after 12½ hours the blood pressure was 150/100, and the fetal heart rate was over 160, labour was permitted to continue for a further 6¾ hours before Caesarean section was advised by Mrs Savage.

3. Mrs Savage gave instructions at 2.45 a.m. for emergency section in an obstructed labour with technical difficulties of delivery inevitable, without herself attending to perform the operation or ensuring that staff of seniority and experience were present and available to undertake it.

6. Generally

1. Taken together, the five cases show a consistent aberration of clinical judgement, thereby exposing the patients to unnecessary and unjustifiable risks.

2. The historical sequence of the five cases indicated a failure to recognise and/or analyse adequately or at all the areas of legitimate concern and/or failure in the light of such analysis to modify her approach accordingly.

3. By her responses to the criticisms made of her conduct of the five cases, Mrs Savage:

   (i) indicates an unwillingness and/or inability to recognise genuine causes for concern affecting patient safety;

   (ii) demonstrates a readiness to avoid and shift personal consultant responsibility for such shortcomings as she is prepared to acknowledge existed;

4. Mrs Savage's conduct and approach as aforesaid was and is not such as meets the standards reasonably required of a senior lecturer at a major teaching hospital, and carries with it the serious risk of:

   (i) confusing junior staff and/or midwives and/or undermining their confidence in, and/or their adherence to reasonable criteria for safe practice;

   (ii) undermining the consistency in standards for safe obstetric practice which such a hosptial ought to teach, establish and maintain;

   (iii) jeopardising the continuity of care which reasonable conformity in such standards between consultants is designed to ensure.

· APPENDIX II ·

General Conclusions of The Panel's Report

We do not agree that the five cases, even if they should properly be taken together, reveal a consistent aberration of clinical judgment. In only one of the cases, AU, did Mrs Savage make a clinical judgment (the suitability of syntocinon in the presence of a breech, a scar and a small pelvis) which went close to the bounds of acceptable practice. We are satisfied that as soon as there were signs that the potential risks in that management could become real rather than theoretical Mrs Savage's advice finally convinced the parents that they should agree to a Caesarean section. We do not agree that, taking the 5 cases together, Mrs Savage's patients were exposed to unnecessary and unjustifiable risks, subject to the qualifications expressed above in respect of the individual cases.

We do not agree that there is any historical sequence of the five cases. Their only connection is that they all took place within a period of about 13 months. In that 13 month period Mrs Savage dealt with many hundreds of other cases, and we have heard no suggestion that complaints could have been made in any of them. In the one other case, that of Y, that we have heard something of, we did not form the view that Mrs Savage acted wrongly in any way. In our view, in all these cases where Mrs Savage has been, to some degree, at fault she has recognised it and tried to analyse it to prevent it happening again. She applied that principle to one case, that of LG, in which the fault was not her own and immediately took steps to see that the error, which had occurred, could not recur.

We do not agree that by defending herself against criticisms which she felt to be unjustified Mrs Savage showed any unwillingness and/or inability to recognise genuine causes for concern affecting patient safety. We recognise that those responsible for the criticisms themselves genuinely felt concern. However, a genuinely felt concern is not necessarily a justified concern. We have indicated in the preceding chapters which concerns we consider to have been justified, and to what extent. We also find that Mrs Savage had an equally genuine concern for patient safety at all times.

We do not agree that Mrs Savage seeks to avoid and shift personal consultant responsibility. She seems to us to recognise that she is broadly responsible for all patients in her care. It does not follow from that, however, that she must necessarily accept personal responsibility and blame for everything which might go wrong in connection with a patient, nor for every mistake which may be made by another person helping to care for the patient. In our view that principle should be applied even more strongly when the issues are not simply about consultant responsibility, but about a consultant's competence, which is a far different and more fundamental thing. A consultant could be personally responsible for mistakes without his competence necessarily being called into question. That principle must also apply where the consultant was not personally responsible for a particular mistake.

We do not agree that Mrs Savage's conduct was, or is, not such as meets the standards reasonably required of a senior lecturer at a major teaching (or any) hospital.

We do not agree that Mrs Savage's conduct and approach carry with them any risk of confusing junior staff and/or midwives. Such persons must understand that in obstetrics, as in all medicine, there is often more than one valid way to deal with a particular situation. We have heard no evidence of sufficient weight that Mrs Savage's criteria for safe practice are unreasonable, nor that Mrs Savage has sought to affect, or even unconsciously affected, any person's adherence to reasonable criteria for safe practice.

We have heard no evidence of sufficient weight to indicate that Mrs Savage's general standards for safe obstetric practice are lower than those of anyone else at the London Hospital. We have heard no evidence to justify the charge that Mrs Savage's conduct (or approach) undermined the consistency of standards in the London Hospital.

We have had no evidence to indicate that any failing of continuity of care as between Mrs Savage and any other consultant can be blamed on Mrs Savage more than any other person.